Veterinary Technician's Handbook of Laboratory Procedures

T0074859

Veterinary Technician's Handbook of Laboratory Procedures

Second Edition

Brianne Bellwood, MSc, RVT, VTS (Clinical Pathology), CCRVN
Alberta Veterinary Technologist Association (ABVTA)
Alberta Veterinary Medical Association (ABVMA)
Academy of Veterinary Clinical Pathology Technicians (AVCPT)

Melissa Andrasik-Catton, RVT, BS
Kansas City Registered Veterinary Technician Association (KCRVTA)
Missouri Veterinary Technician Association (MOVTA)

WILEY Blackwell

Registered Office
John Wiley & Sons, Inc., 111 River Street, Hoboken, NJ 07030, USA

For details of our global editorial offices, customer services, and more information about Wiley products visit us at www.wiley.com.

Wiley also publishes its books in a variety of electronic formats and by print-on-demand. Some content that appears in standard print versions of this book may not be available in other formats.

Library of Congress Cataloging-in-Publication Data
Names: Bellwood, Brianne, author. | Andrasik-Catton, Melissa, author.
Title: Veterinary technician's handbook of laboratory procedures / Brianne
    Bellwood, Melissa Andrasik-Catton.
Description: Second edition. | Hoboken, NJ : Wiley-Blackwell, 2023. |
    Includes bibliographical references and index.
Identifiers: LCCN 2022036458 (print) | LCCN 2022036459 (ebook) | ISBN
    9781119672616 (paperback) | ISBN 9781119672647 (adobe pdf) | ISBN
    9781119672654 (epub) | ISBN 9781119672678 (obook)
Subjects: MESH: Clinical Laboratory Techniques–veterinary | Animal
    Technicians | Handbook
Classification: LCC SF772.6 (print) | LCC SF772.6 (ebook) | NLM SF 772.6
    | DDC 636.089/607-dc23/eng/20221024
LC record available at https://lccn.loc.gov/2022036458
LC ebook record available at https://lccn.loc.gov/2022036459

Cover Design: Wiley
Cover Image: Courtesy of Brianne Bellwood

Set in 10/13pt Interstate-Light by Straive, Pondicherry, India

Printed in Singapore
M105636_151122

Brianne Bellwood:

To my family and friends, whose continued support and encouragement have motivated me to pursue additional endeavors. To my students, past, present, and future, whose enthusiasm and passion for learning inspire me every day.

Melissa Andrasik-Catton:

Foremost, I want to thank my amazing husband and family for their unconditional support of my profession – the many hours spent working ER or teaching and missing family functions, extensive travel for conferences and work, or sitting behind my computer at all hours. I'd like to dedicate this book to two incredible mentors who made me the technician I am today – Dr. Carole Maltby and Dr. Jeff Dennis – two minds that imparted immeasurable knowledge and wisdom to a brain willing to absorb it all. Thanks to all of you, my successes in life are because of you.

Contents

Preface

Laboratory analysis is an essential diagnostic component of veterinary medicine. The skilled veterinary technician plays a vital role in collecting, processing, analyzing, and reporting their findings to the veterinarian. This text is intended to be a helpful guide when performing many common laboratory tests and serves as an excellent companion to full textbooks. The following chapters incorporate discussions on common laboratory equipment: quality control methods, hematology, chemistry, serology, urinalysis, parasitology, microbiology, and cytology.

This new edition has expanded on the topics covered in the first edition and now includes microbiology and serology sections. Additional images help the technician identify microscopic findings and guide them when performing these analyses.

Beneficial characteristics of this handbook, whether used in school or a clinic setting, are:

- Step-by-step procedures.
- Discussions of quality assurance and quality control methods.
- Plenty of reference images.

In contrast to other resources available, this book provides needed information quickly and at a glance.

An accompanying website provides additional resources, case studies, and study tools for students.

Acknowledgements

I would like to thank the Lakeland College Animal Health Technology program team for assistance in providing resources and samples for this book.

-B.B.

I would like to thank Maple Woods Veterinary Technology Program for providing certain resources found in this book.

-M. A.-C.

List of Abbreviations

ACT	Activated clotting time
ALB	Albumin
ALP	Alkaline phosphatase
ALT	Alanine aminotransferase
AMY	Amylase
aPTT	Activated partial thromboplastin time
AST	Aspartate aminotransferase
BA	Bile acids
BAP	Blood agar plate
BMBT	Buccal mucosa bleeding time
BTT	Blue-top tube
BUN	Blood urea nitrogen
Ca	Calcium
CBC	Complete blood count
cELISA	Competitive enzyme-linked immunosorbent assay
CHOL	Cholesterol
CK	Creatine kinase
Cl	Chloride
cPLI	Canine specific pancreatic lipase
CREA	Creatinine
CSF	Cerebrospinal fluid
DTM	Dermatophyte testing media
EDTA	Ethylenediaminetetraacetic acid
ELISA	Enzyme-linked immunosorbent assay
ESA	Enhanced sporulation agar
FNB	Fine-needle biopsy
fPLI	Feline specific pancreatic lipase
GGT	Gamma-glutamyltransferase
GLOB	Globulin
GLU	Glucose
GTT	Green top tube
HCO_3	Bicarbonate
HCT	Hematocrit
HPF	High-power field
K	Potassium
KOH	Potassium hydroxide

LD	Lactate dehydrogenase
LIP	Lipase
LPF	Low-power field
LTT	Lavender-top tube
MAC	MacConkey agar
MCH	Mean corpuscular hemoglobin
MCHC	Mean corpuscular hemoglobin concentration
MCV	Mean corpuscular volume
Mg	Magnesium
MH	Mueller-Hinton
MPV	Mean platelet volume
Na	Sodium
NMB	New methylene blue
P	Phosphorus
PBS	Peripheral blood smear
PCR	Polymerase chain reaction
PCT	Plateletcrit
PCV	Packed cell volume
PLT	Platelet
PT	Prothrombin time
PTH	Parathyroid hormone
QA	Quality assurance
QC	Quality control
RBC	Red blood cell
RDW	Red cell distribution width
RIM	Rapid immunomigration test
RPI	Reticulocyte production index
RTE	Renal tubular epithelial cell
RTT	Red top tube
SDMA	Symmetric dimethylarginine
SOP	Standard operating procedure
SS	*Salmonella-Shigella* agar
SST	Serum separator tube
TBIL	Total bilirubin
TLI	Trypsin-like immunoreactivity
TNCC	Total nucleated cell count
Total T_4	Thyroxine
TP	Total protein
TSA	Trypticase soy agar
TSH	Thyroid stimulating hormone
USG	Urine specific gravity
WBC	White blood cell

About the Companion Website

This book is accompanied by a companion website.

www.wiley.com/go/bellwoodhandbook2

This website includes:

- Case studies provided as PDFs
- PowerPoints of all figures from the book for downloading
- Crossword puzzles and answers as PDFs
- Video of peripheral blood smear technique
- PowerPoints of additional figures for downloading

Chapter 1
Laboratory Equipment

Laboratory equipment

The variety of sophisticated laboratory equipment in a veterinary practice will depend largely on the size and scope of the practice itself. There are several pieces of core equipment that are standard in every practice that performs in-house testing and analysis.

Microscope

Purpose

The microscope is the most important piece of equipment in the veterinary clinic laboratory (Figure 1.1). The microscope is used to review fecal, urine, blood, and cytology samples on a daily basis. Understanding how the microscope functions, how it operates, and how to care for it will improve the reliability of your results and prolong the life of this valuable piece of equipment.

Parts and functions of a compound microscope

(A) **Arm:** Used to carry the microscope.

(B) **Base:** Supports the microscope and houses the light source.

(C) **Oculars (or eyepieces):** The lens of the microscope you look through. The ocular also magnifies the image. The total magnification can be calculated by multiplying the objective power by the ocular power. Oculars come in different magnifications, but 10× magnification is common.

(D) **Diopter adjustment:** The purpose of the diopter adjustment is to correct the differences in vision an individual may have between their left and right eyes.

(E) **Interpupillary adjustment:** This allows the oculars to move closer or further away from one another to match the width of the space between an individual's eyes. When looking through the microscope, one should see only a single field of view. When viewing a sample, always use both eyes. Using one eye can cause eye strain over time.

(F) **Nosepiece:** The nosepiece holds the objective lenses. The objectives are mounted on a rotating turret so they can be moved into place as needed. Most nosepieces can hold up to five objectives.

Veterinary Technician's Handbook of Laboratory Procedures, Second Edition. Brianne Bellwood
and Melissa Andrasik-Catton.
© 2023 John Wiley & Sons, Inc. Published 2023 by John Wiley & Sons, Inc.
Companion website: www.wiley.com/go/bellwoodhandbook2

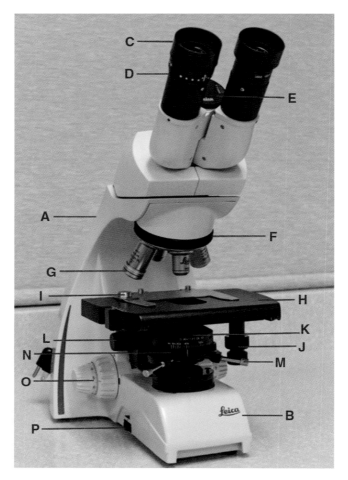

Figure 1.1 Parts of a compound microscope.

(G) **Objective lenses:** The objective lens is the lens closest to the object being viewed, and its function is to magnify the object. Objective lenses are available in many powers, but 4×, 10×, 40×, and 100× are standard. The 4× objective is used mainly for scanning. The 10× objective is considered "low power", 40× is "high power" and the 100× objective is referred to as "oil immersion." When the 10× and 40× objectives are used to view images, the terms "low-power field" (LPF) for 10× and "high-power field" (HPF) for 40× are often used. Once magnified by the objective lens, the image is viewed through the oculars, which magnify it further. Total magnification can be calculated by multiplying the objective power by the ocular lens power.

Example: 10× (ocular lens) × 100× (objective lens) = 1000× total magnification of the specimen

(H) **Stage:** The platform on which the slide or object is placed for viewing.
(I) **Stage brackets:** Spring-loaded brackets, or clips, hold the slide or specimen in place on the stage.

(J) **Stage control knobs:** Located just below the stage are the stage control knobs. These knobs move the slide or specimen either horizontally (*x* axis) or vertically (*y* axis) when it is being viewed.

(K) **Condenser:** The condenser is located under the stage. As light travels from the illuminator, it passes through the condenser, where it is focused and directed at the specimen.

(L) **Condenser control knob:** Allows the condenser to be raised or lowered.

(M) **Condenser centering screws:** These screws center the condenser and, therefore, the beam of light. Generally, they do not need much adjustment unless the microscope is moved or transported frequently.

(N) **Iris diaphragm:** This structure controls the amount of light that reaches the specimen. Opening and closing the iris diaphragm adjusts the diameter of the light beam.

(O) **Coarse and fine focus adjustment knobs:** These knobs bring the object into focus by raising and lowering the stage. Care should be taken when adjusting the stage height. When a higher-power objective is in place (100× objective, for example), there is a risk of raising the stage and slide and hitting the objective lens. This can break the slide and scratch the lens surface.

Coarse adjustment is used for finding focus under low power and adjusting the stage height. Fine adjustment is used for more delicate, high-power adjustments.

(P) **Illuminator:** The illuminator is the light source for the microscope, usually situated in the base. The brightness of the light from the illuminator can be adjusted to suit your preference and the object you are viewing.

Kohler illumination
What is Kohler illumination?
Kohler illumination is a method of adjusting a microscope in order to provide optimal illumination by focusing the light on the specimen. When a microscope is set up in Kohler illumination, specimens will appear clearer and in more detail (Procedure 1.1).

Procedure 1.1   Setting Kohler

Materials
- Specimen slide (need to focus under 10× power)
- Compound microscope.

Procedure
(1) Mount the specimen slide on the stage and focus under 10×.
(2) Close the iris diaphragm completely.
(3) If the ball of light is not in the center, use the condenser centering screws to move it so that it is centered.
(4) Using the condenser adjustment knobs, raise or lower the condenser until the edges of the field become sharp. (See Figures 1.2 and 1.3.)
(5) Open the iris diaphragm until the entire field is illuminated.

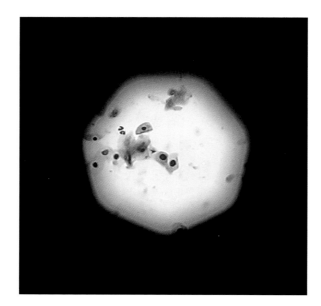

Figure 1.2 Appearance of image prior to setting the condenser. Note the softer edges of unfocused light.

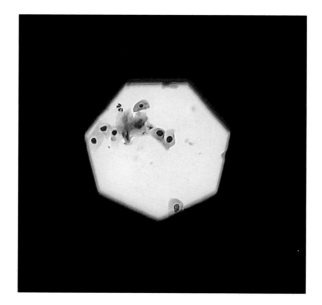

Figure 1.3 Sharpened edges following condenser adjustment.

When should you set/check Kohler?
- During regular microscope maintenance
- After the microscope is moved/transported
- Whenever you suspect objects do not appear as sharp as they could be

Microscope care and maintenance

Routine care and proper maintenance of the microscope will ensure good performance over the years. In addition to this, a properly maintained and clean microscope will always be ready for use at any time (Figure 1.4). Professional cleaning and maintenance should be considered when routine techniques fail to produce optimal performance of the microscope.

Cleaning and maintenance supplies

Dust cover: When not in use, a microscope should be covered to protect it from dust, hair, and any other possible sources of dirt. A dust cover should never be placed over a microscope while the illuminator is still on.

Lens tissue: Lint-free lens tissues are delicate wipes that will not scratch the surface of the oculars or objective. Always ensure that you are using these types of tissues. Never substitute facial tissues or paper towels, as they are too abrasive.

Lens cleaner: Lens cleaning solution assists in removing fingerprints and smudges from lenses and objectives. Apply the lens cleaner to the lens tissue paper and clean/polish the surface.

Compressed-air duster: Using compressed air to rid the microscope of dust particles is far superior to using your own breath and blowing onto the microscope. Compressed air is clean and avoids possible contamination from moisture.

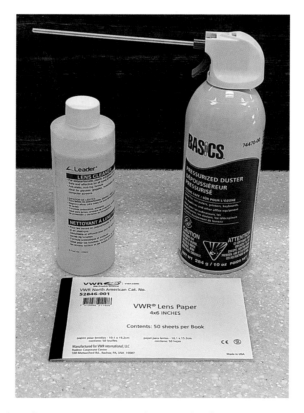

Figure 1.4   Examples of recommended cleaning supplies for the compound microscope.

Microscope cleanup procedure

When the use of the microscope is complete, following proper cleanup procedures will improve the quality of images that are viewed and extend the life of the microscope and its components.

(1) Remove the slide from the stage and dispose of it properly.
(2) Clean any oil residue or sample material that may have contaminated the stage surface.
(3) Lower the stage and move the smallest objective into place.
(4) Clean the objective lens and oculars after every use. The order in which they are cleaned is important. Cleaning the 100× objective first and then moving onto other parts will result in immersion oil being spread onto all other components. Using lens tissue and lens cleaner, begin with cleaning the oculars, then the 4× objective, the 10× objective, 40× objective, and finish with the 100× objective lens.

Maintenance tips

(1) Whenever the microscope is not in use, turn off the illuminator. This will greatly extend the life of the bulb, as well as keeping the temperature down during extended periods of laboratory work.
(2) When cleaning the microscope, use distilled water or lens cleaner. Avoid using other chemicals or solvents, as they may be corrosive to the rubber or lens mounts.
(3) After using immersion oil, clean off any residue immediately. Avoid rotating the 40× objective through immersion oil. If this should occur, immediately clean the 40× objective with lens cleaner before the oil has a chance to dry.
(4) Do not be afraid to use many sheets of lens tissue when cleaning. Use a fresh piece when moving to a different part of the microscope. This avoids tracking dirt/oil/residue to other areas of the microscope.
(5) Store the microscope safely with the stage lowered and the smallest objective in position (4× or 10×). This placement allows the greatest distance between the stage and the objective. If the microscope is bumped, the likelihood of an objective becoming damaged by the stage surface will be greatly minimized.

Centrifuge

Another key component of the veterinary laboratory is the centrifuge. Numerous centrifuge types exist for different purposes, such as those for microhematocrit, fecal, urine, and blood samples. It is not uncommon to use a multifunction centrifuge that can be set to spin at a speed appropriate for the biological sample, with specialized holding devices for each type of sample. The manufacturer's guide should be used for operation, maintenance, and cleaning instructions.

Microhematocrit centrifuge

This centrifuge is used exclusively for spinning down microhematocrit tubes (Figure 1.5). This process is used for determining a patient's packed cell volume (PCV) and can also provide a plasma sample for protein analysis.

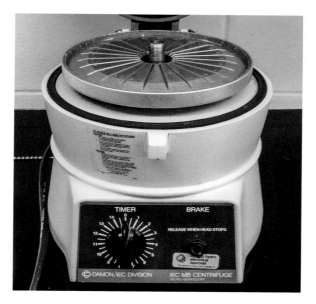

Figure 1.5 Microhematocrit centrifuge.

Clinical centrifuge

Clinical centrifuges are available in two main types: variable-angle centrifuges and fixed-angle centrifuges (Figures 1.6 and 1.7).

The variable-angle centrifuge (also called a horizontal centrifuge) has swinging buckets that hold the specimen tubes. As the centrifugation begins, these buckets swing out horizontally, and the particles within the specimen are pushed to the base of the tube to form the sediment. Once the rotation stops, the buckets return to their upright position. This change of position from horizontal to vertical can result in a slight remixing of the sample. This effect should be taken into consideration when preparing a sample.

The fixed-angle centrifuge has buckets that are in a fixed position, typically about 50°. The specimen tubes are held in this position for the entire centrifugation process.

Refractometer

The purpose of a refractometer is to measure the refractive index of a solution. When a solution (e.g., urine) is measured, light passes through the sample and bends. The angle of this refraction is visualized as a shadow and correlates with the concentration of the solution. Veterinary-specific refractometers are now on the market, allowing minor differences between dog and cat urine specific gravity and total protein values to be discerned. Most are temperature compensated and are intended to be used between 60°F to 100°F. This should be taken into consideration when analyzing samples which have been stored in the refrigerator. They should be allowed to warm to room temperature prior to measuring to maintain accuracy.

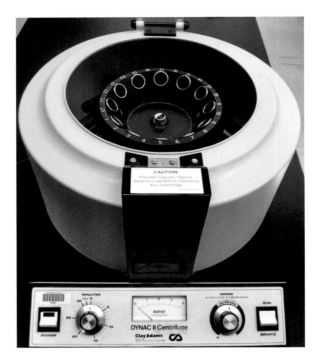

Figure 1.6   Fixed-angle centrifuge.

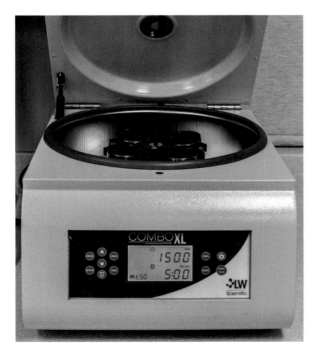

Figure 1.7   Variable-angle centrifuge.

The most common use of a refractometer in veterinary laboratories is to measure urine specific gravity and plasma total protein. Refractometers have built-in scales to measure both, and some brands of refractometers will also possess a refractive index scale. This scale, with the use of an appropriate conversion chart, can be used to measure the concentration of many other solutions (Figures 1.8 and 1.9).

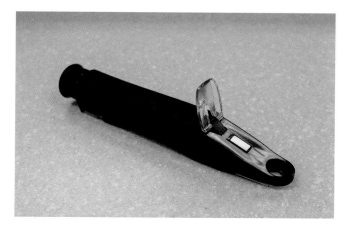

Figure 1.8   Refractometer.

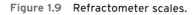

Figure 1.9   Refractometer scales.

Calibration

It is good practice to calibrate the refractometer on a regular basis (daily or weekly, depending on use). This is achieved by applying a large drop of distilled water on the prism and adjusting the blue/white line to read exactly 1.000 on the scale (see Chapter 4, Figure 4.4). Calibration should be done using distilled water at a temperature of 60°F to 100°F. The adjustment knob or screw is variously located on different refractometers; therefore, the manufacturer's guide will need to be consulted.

Incubator

An incubator provides the ability to artificially control the environmental temperature (and humidity, to some extent) for many microbiological procedures. Common in-clinic incubators have a temperature setting and require the placement of a container of water to maintain humidity (Figure 1.10). More expensive incubators can also control the level of humidity as well as the oxygen and carbon dioxide levels; however, these types are not normally seen in general veterinary practices.

In-house analyzers

Chemistry analyzers

There are a wide variety of chemistry analyzers available for veterinary use (Figure 1.11). Most use the principles of photometry to quantify analytes, such as enzymes, proteins, and other constituents in the blood. Electrochemical methods are used to analyze ionic compounds such as electrolytes. These two methods may require the use of two separate analyzers, or they may be combined into one.

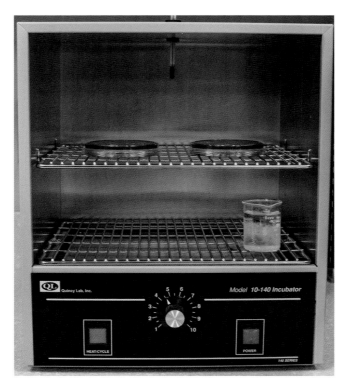

Figure 1.10   Incubator.

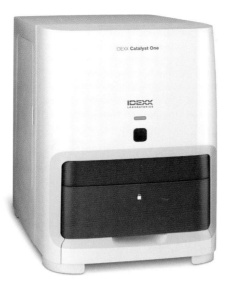

Figure 1.11   IDEXX Catalyst One in-house chemistry analyzer. (Photo provided courtesy of IDEXX Laboratories, Inc.) *Source:* Courtesy of IDEXX Laboratories, Inc.

Another variation among analyzers is the way they facilitate the photometry testing procedure. A sample needs to be added to a substrate to initialize the test. Examples include slides, rotors, and cartridges (Figure 1.12).

Depending upon the analyzer or the analyte being tested, a serum or plasma sample is required. Some analyzers can process whole-blood samples as well. The type of anticoagulant recommended should be confirmed by reviewing the manufacturer recommendations.

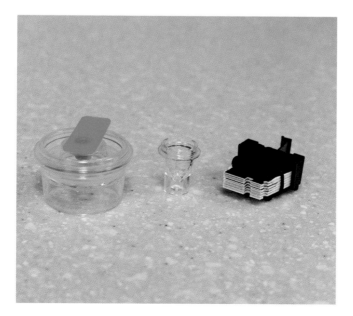

Figure 1.12   Common chemistry testing supplies. Supplies required will depend on the analyzer.

Regardless of the analyzer type chosen, it is important to maintain the equipment according to the manufacturer's recommendations. Regular maintenance and quality control monitoring are essential for ensuring the precision and accuracy of the analyzer. It may also be necessary for complying with the manufacturer's warranty.

Cell counters

As with chemistry analyzers, there are many types of cell counters to choose from (Figure 1.13). There are several different technologies used to quantify cell types, and each has its own advantages and disadvantages. Examples of the technologies used are impedance, laser-based technology, and optical fluorescence. An analyzer may use one or a combination of these technologies to detect and enumerate the cells present in the sample. Most commonly, these analyzers are used for hematology tests (complete blood counts); however, many types can also assess fluids such as peritoneal, thoracic, and synovial fluid samples.

While the analyzers can provide a large amount of information about the patient, it is recommended to follow up with a manual examination of the sample to confirm readings and review morphology of cells.

Coagulation analyzers

In-house coagulation testing (Figure 1.14) is available to screen for coagulation disorders and measure fibrinogen levels. Tests such as prothrombin time (PT), activated partial thromboplastin time (aPTT), and fibrinogen tests can be performed using fresh or citrated whole blood.

As with all analyzers, it is recommended to follow appropriate maintenance and quality control procedures to ensure the accuracy and precision of the equipment.

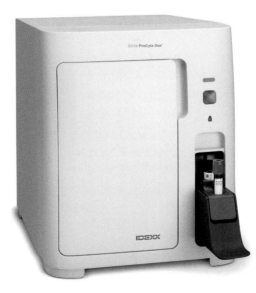

Figure 1.13 IDEXX ProCyte One in-house hematology analyzer. (Photo provided courtesy of IDEXX Laboratories, Inc.) *Source:* Courtesy of IDEXX Laboratories, Inc.

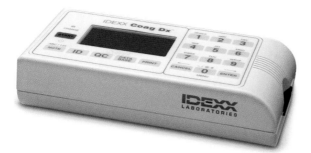

Figure 1.14   IDEXX Coag Dx in-house coagulation analyzer. (Photo provided courtesy of IDEXX Laboratories, Inc.) *Source:* Courtesy of IDEXX Laboratories, Inc.

Quality control and quality assurance

Quality control (QC) consists of actions taken which monitor the performance of the equipment. Internal QC are processes which are "built into" the equipment and are performed automatically (e.g., the quality control on an ELISA [enzyme-linked immunosorbent assay] test kit). External QC processes are not built into the piece of equipment and are required to be performed by veterinary personnel, typically the veterinary technician (e.g., controls used to assess the accuracy of a blood analyzer by comparing generated results to known values). External QC results must be assessed by trained personnel to determine if they are acceptable, and if not, troubleshooting should follow to determine the reason for the failure.

Quality assurance (QA) is defined as procedures which are performed with the goal of minimizing errors and achieving reliable results of diagnostic quality. Examples of QA procedures include proper patient handling, proper sample handling, and following manufacturer's recommendation regarding equipment usage and maintenance. These QA procedures are best to be documented into standard operating procedures (SOPs) to ensure that all veterinary personnel are consistent in their methods. SOPs should be reviewed on a regular basis and updated as needed.

Accuracy, precision, and reliability

"Accuracy," "precision," and "liability" are common terms encountered when assessing a quality control program. Accuracy refers to how close the reading is to the correct value. Precision refers to the reproducibility of a result, and reliability incorporates both the accuracy and precision of a test procedure. The images below (Figures 1.15 to 1.18) are examples of how reliability of a test procedure can be described.

Sources of error

If a quality control procedure fails, troubleshooting should be done to determine the cause. A number of factors can influence the reliability of a test method, many of which are human error; however, the possibility of equipment malfunction should not be overlooked.

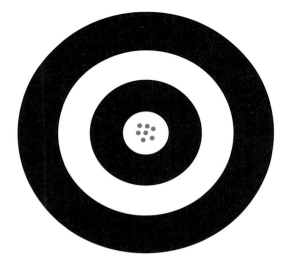

Figure 1.15   High accuracy, high precision.

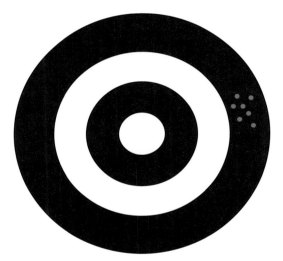

Figure 1.16   Low accuracy, high precision.

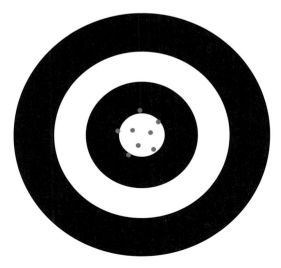

Figure 1.17   High accuracy, low precision.

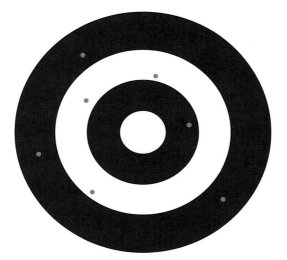

Figure 1.18   Low accuracy, low precision.

Preanalytic variables
Preanalytic variables include any variations from the standard which occur prior to testing. Biologic variables are related to the patient; examples include breed and age. These variables cannot be controlled; however, if comprehensive patient information is included with the test results, the veterinarian can more accurately interpret the results. Other biologic variables can be controlled and should be minimized whenever possible. An example would be having a patient fast prior to sampling. Nonbiologic variables are not related to the patient and could include mislabeling of a sample or sample collection and handling errors. Efforts should be made to avoid these by following clinic SOPs and educating the veterinary personnel on the importance of these methods.

Analytic variables
Analytic variables are related to the instrument measurement itself. These errors can arise from inadequate maintenance of equipment or using outdated reagents. Such errors tend to reveal themselves gradually, and a proper QC program should highlight any trends and identify issues early.

Postanalytic variables
Postanalytic variables occur following sample processing and include the incorrect reporting or recording of results.

Chapter 2

Hematology and Coagulation Testing

Performing a complete blood count (CBC) involves the use of manual and automated methods to examine the numbers and characteristics of the red blood cell (RBC), white blood cell (WBC), and platelet populations. The robustness and accuracy of these tests are dependent on the analyzer used and the skill of the veterinary technician performing the examination.

Coagulation testing involves the assessment of the components for hemostasis, such as platelets, platelet factors, and coagulation factors. Point-of-care analyzers and manual tests can be used to establish coagulation profiles in clinics, with additional testing conducted at external laboratories.

Peripheral blood smears

Peripheral blood smear (PBS) examination is an essential component of the CBC. Smears are utilized to examine and count cell types, evaluate cellular morphology, and validate automated analyzer results. The quality of the smear directly affects the accuracy of the results; therefore, creating a well-made diagnostic blood smear is crucial.

The blood smear is made using the wedge smear technique (Figure 2.1), with the goal being to obtain an adequate monolayer where the cells are evenly distributed (not overlapping or spread too far apart) and their morphologies can be accurately examined (Procedure 2.1).

Procedure 2.1   Preparing a peripheral blood smear

Materials
- Well-mixed anticoagulated whole blood
  If possible, the use of a drop of blood directly from the patient to the slide will reduce the potential for dilution, clumping and artifact influences on your PBS
- Glass microscope slides
- Capillary tube
- Lens tissue

Veterinary Technician's Handbook of Laboratory Procedures, Second Edition. Brianne Bellwood and Melissa Andrasik-Catton.
© 2023 John Wiley & Sons, Inc. Published 2023 by John Wiley & Sons, Inc.
Companion website: www.wiley.com/go/bellwoodhandbook2

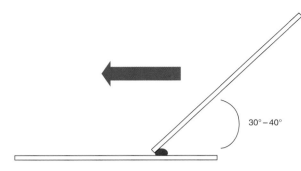

30°–40°

Figure 2.1 Technique for preparing a peripheral blood smear (*see demo video on accompanying website*).

Procedure

(1) It is important to begin with two clean, dust-free microscope slides. If slides are dirty or dusty, polish them using lint-free lens tissue. Avoid touching the glass with your fingers.
(2) After inverting the whole blood tube several times gently, obtain a small amount using the capillary tube. If blood is not well mixed, cells will begin to settle, causing the cell distribution on your PBS to be inaccurate.
(3) Using the capillary tube, place a small drop of blood (2–3 mm) at the end of your slide.
(4) The second slide is used as a "spreader" slide and should be held at a 30°–40° angle (see Figure 2.1).
(5) Using a thumb and forefinger, anchor the bottom slide to the counter and back the spreader slide into the blood drop.
(6) Pause at the blood drop briefly, allowing the blood drop to flow across the edge of the spreader slide, and in a smooth fluid motion, advance the spreader slide to the end.
(7) Be sure not to change your angle or lift the spreader slide off of the bottom slide (see Table 2.1 for additional points).

Characteristics of a good smear

- Covers 3/4 of the slide
- Symmetrical, bullet shape
- No tails or ridges
- Microscopically, should have an even distribution of cells within the monolayer (Figure 2.2) displaying even cell distribution)

Blood smears are most commonly stained with the Romanowsky-type stain (Procedure 2.2), which allows adequate visualization of cell structures and morphologies (see Figure 7.13 in chapter 7). New methylene blue stains can also be used in identifying reticulocytes and Heinz bodies.

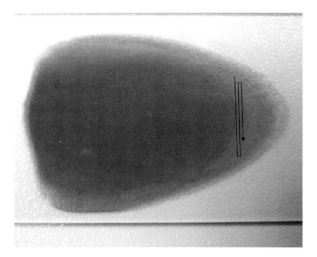

Figure 2.2 Example of a diagnostic quality PBS. Note the highlighted monolayer, or "read area" of the slide. Microscopically, the cells should have an even distribution in this area of the slide.

Procedure 2.2   Diff-Quik staining of a blood smear

(1) Before staining, ensure the smear is completely dry.
(2) Dip the slide, submerging the entire blood smear into the fixative 5 times, for 1 second each. Drain the excess.
(3) Dip the slide into the stain 1, five times, for one second each. Drain the excess.
(4) Dip the slide into the stain 2, five times, for one second each. Drain the excess.
(5) Rinse with distilled water.
(6) Allow to air dry completely before examining the slide.

The timing of each step may be adjusted depending on the sample type, sample thickness and desired staining outcome.

Troubleshooting

Creating a diagnostic quality blood smear takes practice, and the technician should be aware that slight modifications in technique will be required depending on the patient sample (Table 2.1). For example, a dehydrated patient will have a blood consistency that is thicker, whereas an anemic patient will have a blood consistency which is thinner. Thicker blood samples spread more slowly, whereas thinner samples spread faster. Adjusting the spreading speed and the length of the "pause" at the blood drop are necessary modifications to the technique.

Table 2.1 Common errors in preparing a blood smear

Error	Description	Considerations and tips
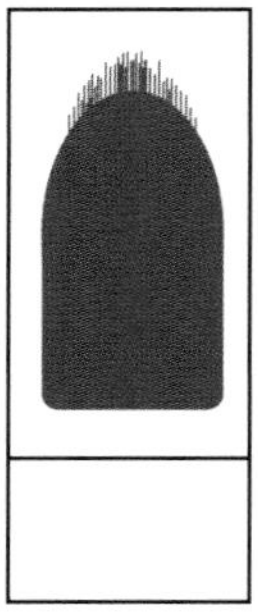 Figure 2.3 "Tails" present on the feathered edge.	Tails	Causes Lifting the spreader slide up at the end of the spreading motion. Debris present on the slide. Cell clumps present in the sample. Poor quality slides. Consequence Uneven distribution of cells within the monolayer. Recommendations Ensure the spreader slide remains in contact for the length of the bottom slide. Wipe slides prior to making a smear and examine their quality. Redraw a new sample if clumping has occurred due to a sample collection and handling error.
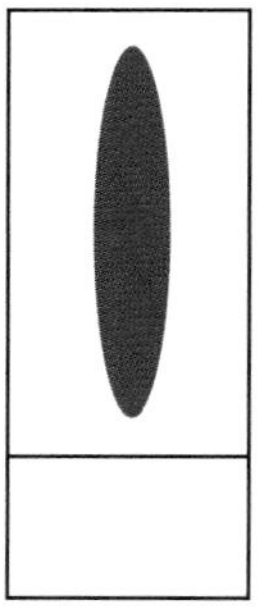 Figure 2.4 Long and narrow.	Long and narrow	This results when the blood is spread too soon before it has had the chance to spread along the edge of the spreader slide. Consequence The shape of the smear doesn't provide a true monolayer which makes the slide difficult to navigate microscopically. Recommendations Pause longer when backing into the drop. Slow your speed slightly when moving the spreader slide forward.
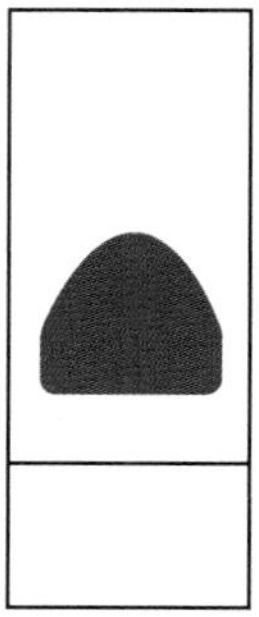 Figure 2.5 Short and wide.	Short and wide	If the spreader slide is held at an angle greater than 30°, the blood may not be pushed out over the length of the slide. Consequence Thick smear with a narrow monolayer making cell identification difficult. Recommendations Lower the angle of the spreader slide

Table 2.1 (*Continued*)

Error	Description	Considerations and tips
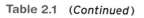Figure 2.6 Square.	Square	A square-shaped smear can be seen when moving forward too slowly. Consequence Overly large, expanded monolayer where the cell distribution can be compromised. Recommendations Increase the forward motion speed of the spreader slide
Figure 2.7 Half-smear.	Half-bullet	A half-smear is the result of uneven pressure and contact from the spreader slide. Consequence The monolayer counting area is reduced by half. Recommendations To ensure even right-to-left pressure of the spreader slide, standing (vs. sitting) while making the smear may help.
Figure 2.8 Holes.	Holes	A smear filled with holes can result when: The slide has dirty or a greasy film from fingerprints or immersion oil. The sample was collected from a patient who recently ate, resulting in the presence of lipids in the blood. Consequence Void areas within the monolayer Recommendations Ensure that slides and work area are clean. If possible, the patient should fast prior to blood collection.

The erythrogram—RBC evaluations

Packed cell volume

It is important to note that packed cell volume (PCV) and hematocrit are often used interchangeably; however, they are measured in different manners and have different sources of error. Here, we discuss the manual packed cell volume method of estimating the portion of whole blood that is composed of red blood cells (Procedure 2.3).

Procedure 2.3 Preparing a packed cell volume test

Materials
- Well-mixed, anticoagulated whole blood
- Tube sealant
- Reader card
- Centrifuge
- Capillary tubes

Procedure
(1) Begin with well-mixed, anticoagulated blood.
(2) Fill two capillary tubes 3/4 full with blood, and seal one end with clay. Filling a second tube serves two purposes:
  - Serves as a counterbalance for centrifugation
  - Serves as a quality control to ensure accuracy.
(3) Place tubes in the groves of the centrifuge, directly across from one another, with the clay pointing towards the outside (see Figure 2.9).
(4) Close centrifuge lid(s).

Speed: 10,000 rpm*
Time: 5 minutes*
*General recommendation. Species and unit may require different speed and time.

Reading the PCV
(1) After centrifugation, the blood in the microhematocrit tubes is separated into three layers: the plasma layer, the buffy coat layer, and the red cell layer (see Figure 2.10).
(2) Using a reader card, align the top of the plasma layer with the 100 line and the bottom of the red cell layer (between the red cells and the top of the clay) with the 0 (see Figure 2.11).
(3) Measurement is taken at the top of the red cell layer where the red cells and buffy coat meet and is expressed as a percentage.
(4) Repeat for tube no. 2.
(5) For quality control purposes, each tube reading should be within one percentage point of the average of the two tubes (e.g., one is 55% and the other is 57%; average is 56%. Both tubes are 1% away from 56%).
(6) Measurement should be taken within 10 minutes of centrifugation to avoid expansion of the packed cell layers.

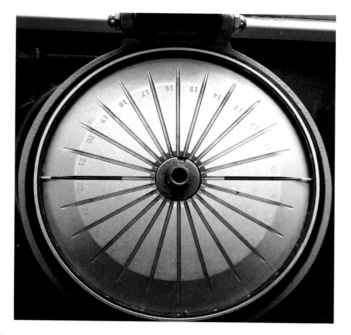

Figure 2.9   Proper placement of PCV tubes into a microhematocrit centrifuge. The tubes are balanced, and the sealant is to the outside.

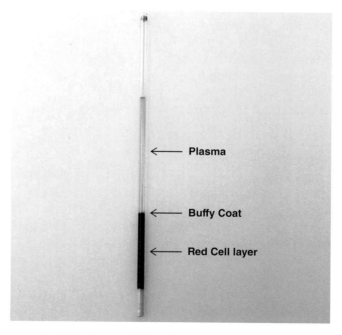

Figure 2.10   Layers of a PCV after centrifugation.

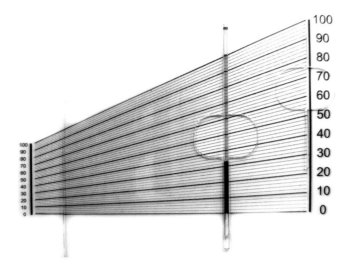

Figure 2.11 Proper alignment of the PCV tube for reading. Note the bottom of the red cell layer is aligned with 0 and the top of the plasma is at 100.

Sources of error

- Excessive anticoagulant in the blood sample
- Using poorly mixed blood
- Incorrect speed and time for the type of centrifuge
- Misalignment of tubes with the reader card
- Including the buffy coat layer in the PCV measurement
- Allowing the tubes to sit for more than 5 minutes prior to reading. The layers will begin to slant, making reading difficult.

Tip: **The hemoglobin value of a patient can be estimated by dividing the PCV reading by 3.**

Plasma evaluation

Total protein (total serum protein) can be assessed by utilizing the plasma portion of the PCV tube. One of the capillary tubes can be broken above the buffy coat, and the plasma (liquid) can be placed on a refractometer to determine the protein concentration. Depending on your type of refractometer, you will read the TP, SP, or TS column and report the number in grams per deciliter (g/dL) (or g/100 mL).

The color of plasma can yield information about the patient's health. Below are plasma colors and associated disorders.

Clear or light straw-yellow: Normal
Deep yellow: Icteric; liver, or hemolytic disorders (horses naturally have very deep yellow plasma)
Red: Hemolyzed; artificial from poor blood collection technique or hemolytic disorders

Milky: Lipemic; artificial due to recent meal or high cholesterol/triglycerides, which may be due to liver or pancreatic issues.

A combination of these can be seen in samples from patients with multiple abnormalities.

Red blood cell count

Procedure 2.4   Red blood cell count

Materials
- Anticoagulated whole blood
- Isotonic dilution fluid at 1:200 ratio (e.g., Ery-TIC test kit, Bioanalytic GmbH, Germany)
- Improved Neubauer hemocytometer (see Figure 2.12)
- Coverslip (specific for a hemocytometer)
- Microscope with 40× lens objective
- Cell counter

Procedure
(1) Follow instructions of manufacturer of dilution medium to properly mix the blood sample.
(2) Place the clean, hemocytometer-specific coverslip on top of the hemocytometer.
(3) Flood one side of the hemocytometer counting chamber using capillary action.
(4) Count the RBCs within five group squares (see Figure 2.13).
(5) Repeat this procedure on the second side of the hemocytometer.
(6) Calculate totals for side 1 and side 2 of the hemocytometer grid and average.

Calculations
RBC determination should be made using the average between side 1 and side 2.

QC
Each side's total should be within 10% of the average before the calculation below is used.

$$\frac{average \times 10}{1000} = \underline{\qquad} \times 10^6/\mu L$$

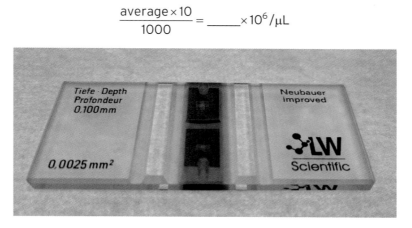

Figure 2.12   Improved Neubauer hemocytometer.

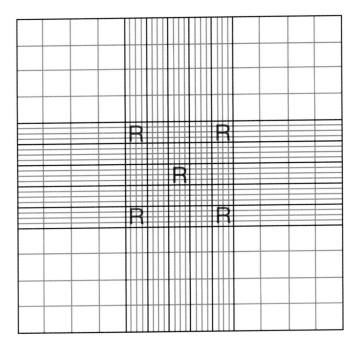

Figure 2.13   Red blood cell counting area (R).

Sources of error
- Improper mixing of whole blood
- Improper filling of commercial dilution device or improper mixing prior to use
- Incomplete filling or overfilling of the hemocytometer chamber
- Using a dirty hemocytometer, which can cause difficulty with differentiating between RBCs and debris.

RBC indices

Calculating the RBC indices can be a useful tool when examining cases of anemia. They can give insight to the size and hemoglobin concentration of the average RBC in the patient's sample. They are often used to determine the type of anemia. These are provided when a CBC analyzer is used.

Information required
- Packed cell volume (L/L)
- Hemoglobin concentration (g/L)
- RBC count (10^6/μL).

Mean corpuscular volume
Being an indicator of volume, mean corpuscular volume (MCV) can provide information regarding the size of the average RBC in a sample.

$$\frac{\text{packed cell volume} \left(\text{L/L} \right)}{\text{RBC count} \left(10^6/\text{μL} \right)} \times 1000 = \underline{\qquad} \text{fL}$$

Interpretation

Value lower than normal = microcytic: red cells are smaller than normal for that species.

Value higher than normal = macrocytic: red cells are larger than normal for that species.

Mean corpuscular hemoglobin

Mean corpuscular hemoglobin (MCH) can provide information regarding the weight of hemoglobin within the average RBC.

$$\frac{\text{hemoglobin } (g/L)}{\text{RBC count } (10^6/\mu L)} = \underline{\hspace{1cm}} pg$$

Interpretation

Values lower than normal = red cells contain less than the average weight of hemoglobin for that species.

Values higher than normal = red cells contain more than the average weight of hemoglobin for that species.

Mean corpuscular hemoglobin concentration

Mean corpuscular hemoglobin concentration (MCHC) provides information regarding the concentration of hemoglobin within the average RBC. MCHC takes into account the amount of hemoglobin in proportion to the size of the average red cell.

$$\frac{\text{hemoglobin } (g/L)}{\text{packed cell volume } (L/L)} = \underline{\hspace{1cm}} g/L$$

Interpretation

Value lower than normal = hypochromic: average red cell contains a lower concentration of hemoglobin for that species

Value higher than normal = average red cell contains a higher concentration of hemoglobin for that species.

Red cell distribution width

Red cell distribution width (RDW) is an analyzer-generated value which indicates the variation of red cell volume in the sample. An increased RDW suggests a greater degree of anisocytosis, meaning that small and large RBCs are present. A normal RDW indicates that the red cells in the sample are fairly uniform in size.

Reticulocyte count

Performing a reticulocyte count is indicated in cases of anemia, to determine whether the anemia is regenerative or nonregenerative. A reticulocyte count should be performed on every anemic patient (except for horses, which do not release reticulocytes into circulation) (Procedure 2.5).

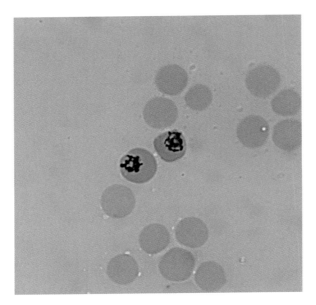

Figure 2.14   Blood smear stained with new methylene blue displaying 2 aggregate reticulocytes.

Note: Two forms of reticulocytes exist: punctate and aggregate (Figure 2.14). In cats, only the aggregate forms should be counted.

Procedure 2.5   Manual reticulocyte count

Materials
- New methylene blue (NMB) stain
- Whole blood
- Microscope slides
- Sterile red-top tube
- Microscope with 100× objective
- Cell counter

Procedure
Before preparing slides, the NMB stain should be filtered by pouring the stain through a layer of filter paper. This process will minimize artifacts such as stain precipitate, which may be falsely recorded as reticulocytes.

(1) Mix equal parts whole blood with filtered NMB stain in a sterile red-top tube.
(2) Allow mixture to sit for 15–20 minutes, gently mixing every 5 minutes.
(3) Prepare two smears as you would for a PBS and allow to air dry.
(4) Reticulocyte counts are made by recording the number of reticulocytes seen per 500 RBCs under 1000× magnification.
(5) Repeat this process on smear no. 2.

QC
Smear 1 and smear 2 totals should be within 20% of each other before calculations are made.

Relative reticulocyte percentage

$$\frac{total\,(side\,1+\,side\,2)}{1000}\times100 = \underline{\quad\quad}\%$$

Absolute reticulocyte count

$$\frac{relative\,(\%)}{100}\times RBC\,count\,(10^6/\mu L)\times1000 = \underline{\quad\quad}\times10^3/\mu L$$

Corrected reticulocyte percentage
In cases of anemia, a reticulocyte percentage can be misleading, since the total number of RBCs is decreased. Correcting your reticulocyte percentage takes into account the decreased total mature RBC numbers circulating in the anemic patient.

$$relative\,(\%)\times\frac{observed\,PCV}{normal\,species\,PCV} = \underline{\quad\quad}\%$$

For dogs: A PCV of 45% is used in the equation.
For cats: A PCV of 35% is used in the equation.

Reticulocyte production index
Prematurely released reticulocytes have a longer lifespan than mature erythrocytes. Calculating the reticulocyte production index (RPI) accounts for this extended survival time and gives insight into whether the regenerative response to anemia is adequate (Tables 2.2 and 2.3).

$$RPI = \frac{corrected\,reticulocyte\,(\%)}{retic\,maturation\,time\,factor}$$

For example:
Corrected reticulocyte % = 5%
Patient's PCV = 15% (maturation time factor = 2.5).

$$RPI = \frac{5}{2.5} = 2$$

Table 2.2 Reticulocyte maturation time factor

Patient PCV	Maturation time factor
45%	1
35%	1.4
25%	2
15%	2.5

Table 2.3   Reticulocyte production index (RPI) interpretation for dogs

RPI < 1	Nonregenerative anemia
RPI 1–2	Responsive bone marrow
RPI > 2	Accelerated erythropoiesis
RPI ≥ 3	Significant regeneration

RBC morphology

Chromasia (cell color)

Table 2.4   Chromasia (cell color)

Erythrocyte characteristic	Description	Image/description
Normochromasia	The expected coloring for a typical mammalian erythrocyte is a buffy pink. Note: Adhering to standard staining technique will ensure reproducible results.	The amount of central pallor expected varies between species and is correlated with a discoid-shaped erythrocyte.
Hypochromasia	A decrease in the amount of expected coloring and increased amount of central pallor for that species. Associated with a decreased amount of hemoglobin and is commonly seen in iron-deficiency anemia. A decreased MCHC is also seen with hypochromasia.	Figure 2.15 Hypochromatic erythrocytes (arrows). Note the increased central pallor of the cell.
Polychromasia	Erythrocytes stain a more blue-purple color and may also be larger in size. Polychromasia is associated with younger cells and the color variation is due to the presence of ribosomes. Staining these cells with New Methylene Blue (NMB) allows for better identification of these remnants confirming the cell is a reticulocyte.	Figure 2.16 Polychromatic erythrocytes (arrows).

Table 2.4 (*Continued*)

Erythrocyte characteristic	Description	Image/description
Hyperchromasia (not considered an official coloration term – related to the MCHC)	An increased MCHC can be produced in instances of hemolysis and Heinz bodies. While an increased MCHC can suggest an increase in hemoglobin in the cell, true hyperchromasia likely does not exist.	Spherocytes can have the appearance of "hyperchromasia" as well as microcytic, however this is due to a change in shape from a typical discoid form to a spherical form (see Figure 2.28).

Anisocytosis (cell size)

Table 2.5 Anisocytosis (cell size)

Erythrocyte characteristic	Description	Image/examples
Normocytic	Typical size varies among species and is measured in μm across the diameter of the cell.	Dogs have a typical size of 7 μm, whereas sheep are smaller (5 μm)
Macrocytic	Increased diameter of the erythrocyte. Increased MCV is also seen.	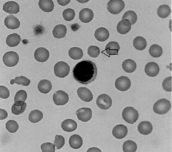 Figure 2.17 Macrocyte (arrow).
Microcytic	Decreased diameter of the erythrocyte. Decreased MCV is also seen.	Figure 2.18 Microcyte (arrow).

Poikilocytosis (cell shape)

"Poikilocytosis" is a general term describing abnormal erythrocyte shape. Subtypes of abnormal shapes can be clinically significant but may also reflect artifactual changes.

Table 2.6   Poikilocytosis (cell shape)

Type of poikilocytosis	Description	Image/examples
Acanthocyte (spur cell)	Multiple blunt, irregular projections extending from the cell. Associated with: Hepatic diseases DIC Hemangiosarcoma Healthy cattle	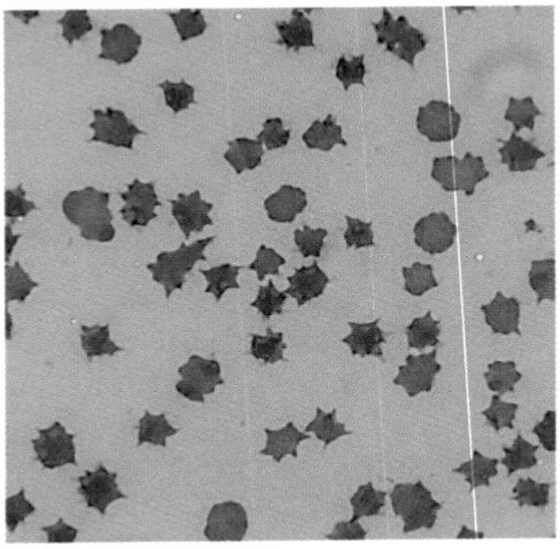 Figure 2.19 Acanthocytes.
Keratocyte (blister cell)	Cells possess a blister-like vesicle on the periphery. This blister may have ruptured and appear as horn-shaped projections. Associated with: Oxidative injury (along with Heinz bodies) Fragmentation injury (along with schistocytes) Hepatic disease	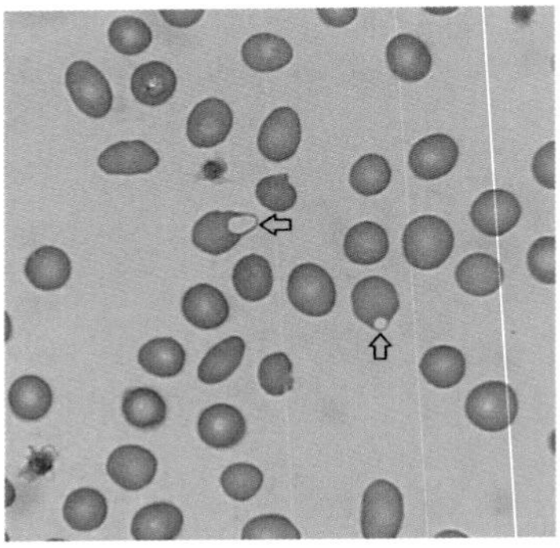 Figure 2.20 Keratocyte (arrows).
Codocytes (leptocytes, target cells)	A "bullseye" shape to the cell caused by a central deposit of hemoglobin. Associated with: Iron deficiency anemia Cell membrane disorder Hepatic disease	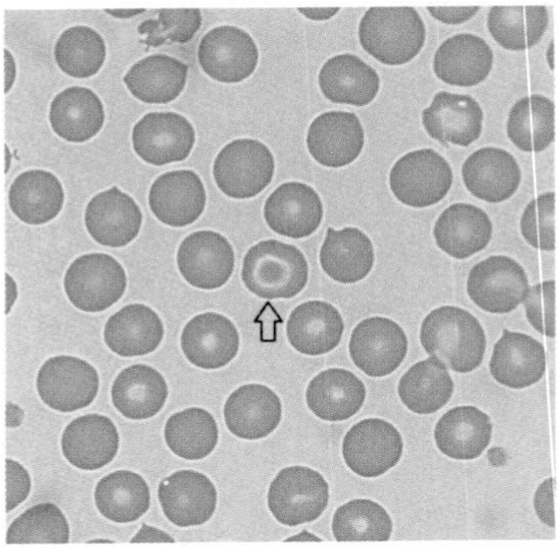 Figure 2.21 Codocyte (arrow).

Table 2.6 (*Continued*)

Type of poikilocytosis	Description	Image/examples
Dacrocytes (teardrop cells)	Teardrop shaped RBCs. Elongated cells have one pointed end. Associated with: Bone marrow disorders Iron deficiency in ruminants	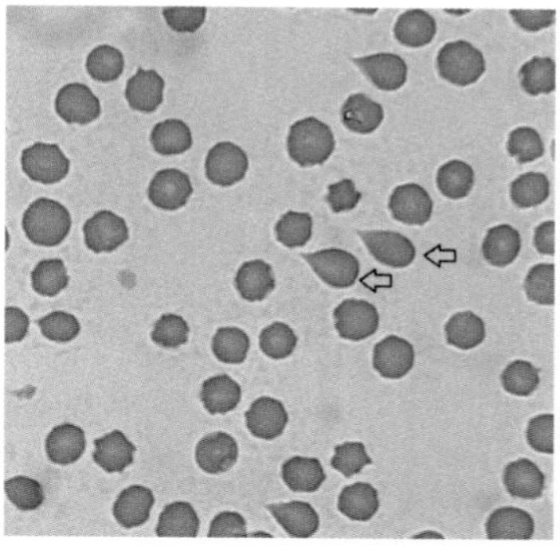 Figure 2.22 Dacrocyte (arrow).
Drepanocyte (sickle cell)	Sickle-shaped erythrocytes. Seen in certain breeds of deer, antelope, sheep and goats.	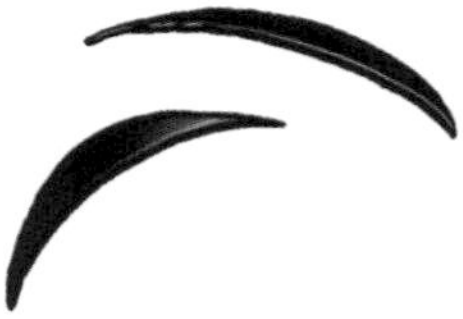 Figure 2.23 Drawing of the typical shape of a drepanocyte.
Eccentrocyte	One side of the erythrocyte is colorless or appears to have a void. Associated with: Oxidative substances (along with Heinz bodies) Hemolytic diseases	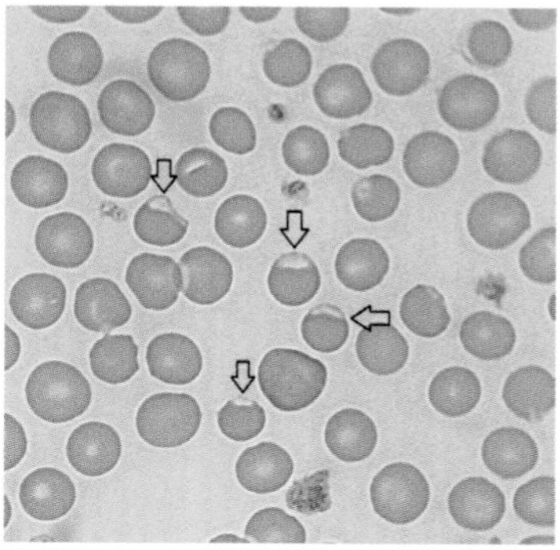 Figure 2.24 Eccentrocyte (arrows).

(*Continued*)

Table 2.6 (*Continued*)

Type of poikilocytosis	Description	Image/examples
Echinocyte (burr cell)	Cells possess small, spiculated, evenly spaced projections. Associated with: Renal disease Snake bite envenomation Frequently seen as an artifact (crenation)	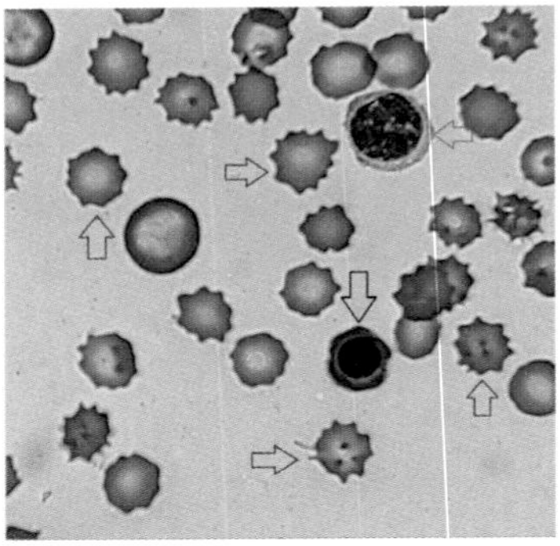 Figure 2.25 Multiple echinocytes (red arrows). Also shown is a nucleated erythrocyte (black arrow) and a lymphocyte (blue arrow).
Elliptocyte (ovalocyte)	Oval or elongated erythrocytes. Normal finding in camelid species and nonmammals. Associated with: Hepatic disorders Hereditary disorders in dogs	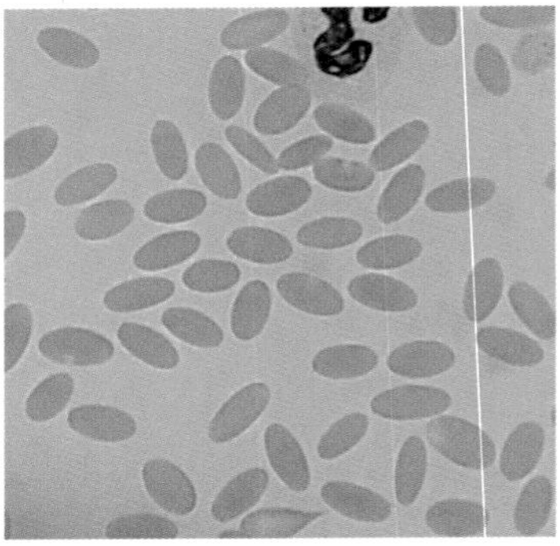 Figure 2.26 Elliptocytes seen in a camelid sample.
Schistocytes	Erythrocyte fragments caused by mechanical injury to the cell. Associated with conditions which cause roughening of the vasculature: DIC Glomerular disease Hemangiosarcoma	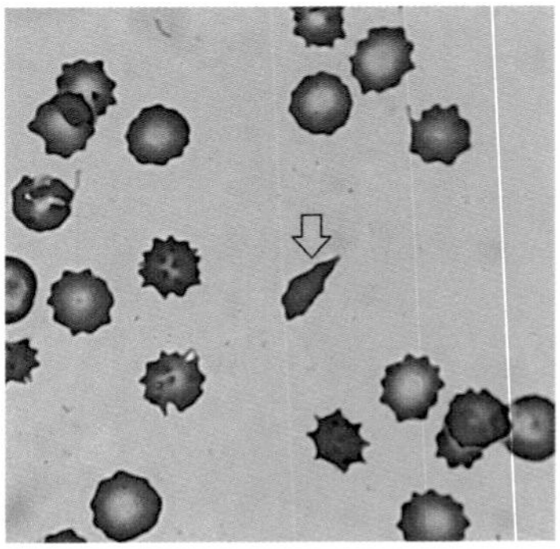 Figure 2.27 Schistocyte (arrow).

Table 2.6 *(Continued)*

Type of poikilocytosis	Description	Image/examples
Spherocyte	Erythrocytes are a spherical shape, no longer a discoid shape and have lost their central pallor. Appear smaller and stain more darkly than other RBCs. Associated with: Immune mediated hemolytic anemia (IMHA) Transfused RBCs	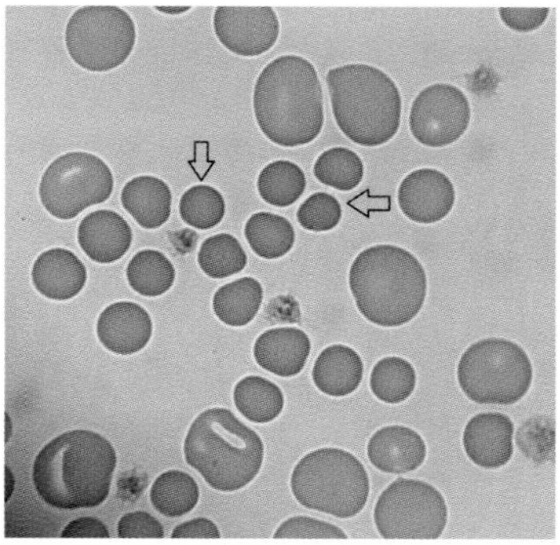 Figure 2.28 Spherocytes (arrows).
Stomatocytes	Erythrocytes with an elongated central pallor which appears as a "mouth-like" area. Associated with: Metabolic disorder Hereditary defect in dogs	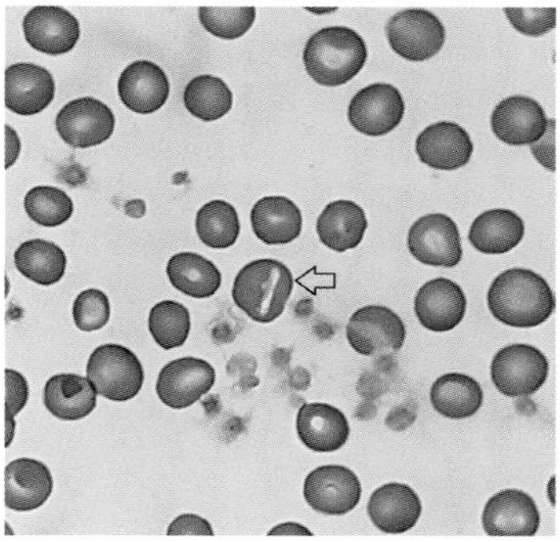 Figure 2.29 Stomatocyte (arrow).

Cell inclusions

Cell inclusions may be confused with artifacts; however, it should be noted that these inclusions are on the same plane of focus as the cell, whereas artifacts would not be. Focusing in and out slightly will make this apparent.

Table 2.7   Cell Inclusions

Erythrocyte characteristic	Description	Image/example(s)
Basophilic stippling	Appear as small blue granules within the RBC. Associated with lead poisoning and a bone marrow regenerative response.	Figure 2.30 Basophilic stippling (arrow).
Heinz bodies	Appear as a singular "bud" protrusion on the exterior of the cell. Associated with oxidative injury which causes a denaturing of the hemoglobin molecule. Examples: acetaminophen in cats; onion, acetaminophen and other oxidative substances in dogs. Can be seen in low numbers in healthy cats. Associated with hemolytic anemia. Staining with NMB will allow Heinz bodies to be easily identified.	Figure 2.31 Heinz body (arrow). Figure 2.32 Heinz bodies (arrows). Stained with new methylene blue.

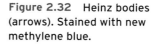

Table 2.7 (Continued)

Erythrocyte characteristic	Description	Image/example(s)
Howell Jolly body	Appear as a singular, dark purple round inclusion within the cell. HJB are remnants of nuclear chromatin and are seen in instances of regeneration. HJB are also seen in patients with a splenectomy.	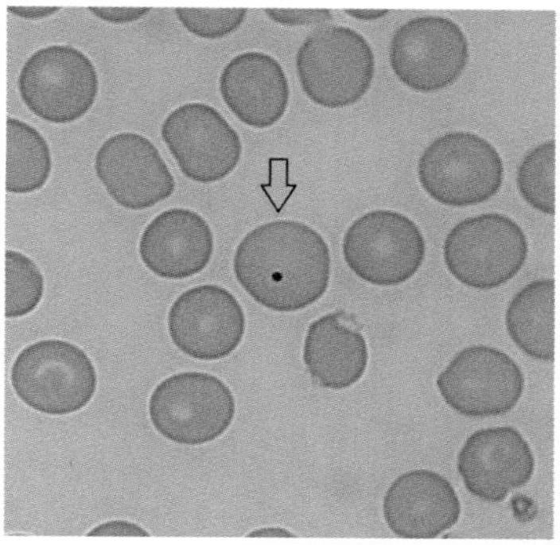 Figure 2.33 Howell-Jolly body (arrow).
Nucleated erythrocytes	RBCs contain a nucleus and display a polychromatic cytoplasm. The appearance of the nucleus will vary depending on the stage of the immature erythrocyte (typically rubricyte or metarubricyte) Associated with bone marrow response and early release of immature erythrocytes.	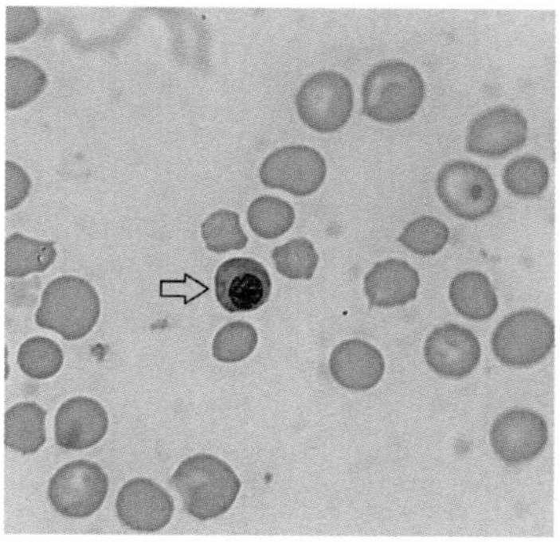 Figure 2.34 Nucleated erythrocyte (NRBC) (arrow).
Siderotic granules	Can be seen with toxic lead poisoning and hemolytic anemia.	Blue-colored iron-containing granules present on the edge of the RBC.

Infectious agents

Table 2.8   Infectious agents

Agent	Description	Image/examples
Anaplasma spp.	Not all species are pathogenic. *Anaplasma* spp. are primarily transmitted through a tick bite. *Anaplasma marginale* — Bovine (infects RBCs) *Anaplasma ovis* — Sheep, goats (infects RBCs; nonpathogenic) *Anaplasma phagocytophilum* (formerly *Ehrlichia equi*) — Horses, dogs, cats, camelids, and humans (infects neutrophils and eosinophils) *Anaplasma platys* (formerly *Ehrlichia platys*) — Dogs (infects platelets)	Multiple small, round, purple, intracellular bacteria.
Babesia spp. and *Theilaria* spp.	Appear as round/oval or teardrop shaped inclusions (based on species) that stain colorless to light-blue. These protozoa are tick-borne and transmitted via a tick bite. Recovered animals often become asymptomatic carriers. *Babesia canis* and *Babesia gibsoni* — Dogs *Babesia felis* — Cats *Babesia caballi* and *Theileria equi* — Horses *Babesia bigemina* and *Babesia bovis* — Cattle *Babesia ovis* and *Babesia motasi* — Sheep	 Figure 2.35 *Babesia canis* (left) and *Babesia gibsoni* (right) present on a canine blood film. (From Thrall MA, Weiser G, Allison RW, and Campbell TW (ed.), *Veterinary Hematology and Clinical Chemistry*, 2nd ed., Ames: Blackwell Publishing, 2012). *Source:* From Thrall et al., (2012), John Wiley & Sons.

Table 2.8 (*Continued*)

Agent	Description	Image/examples
Cytauxzoon felis	Ring-shaped intracellular protozoan of cats.	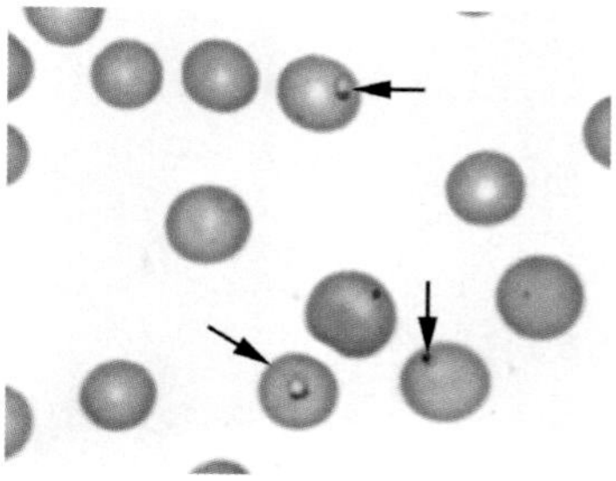 Figure 2.36 *Cytauxzoon* organisms on a feline blood film. (From Thrall MA, Weiser G, Allison RW, and Campbell TW (ed.), *Veterinary Hematology and Clinical Chemistry*, 2nd ed., Blackwell Publishing, Ames, IA, 2012). *Source:* From Thrall et al., (2012), John Wiley & Sons.
Distemper bodies	Viral particles seen during the viremic stage of the canine distemper virus; however, their presence in the blood is transient. Inclusions can be seen in erythrocytes and leukocytes.	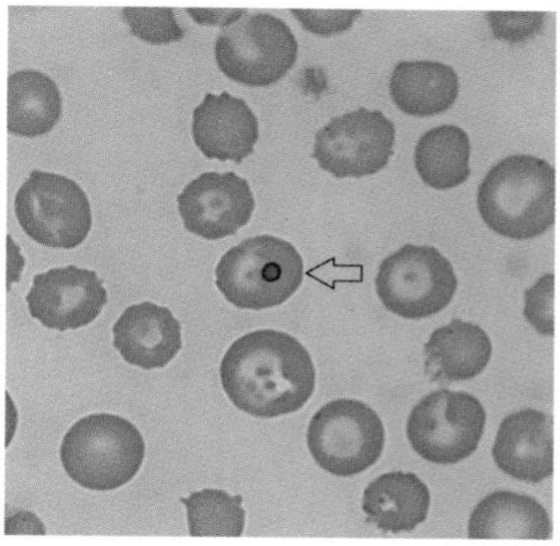 Figure 2.37 Distemper body inclusion.
Mycoplasma spp.	Mycoplasma bacteria appear as small, dark staining round, ring-shaped, or rod-shaped organisms. They appear on the edges or on the surface of the RBC.	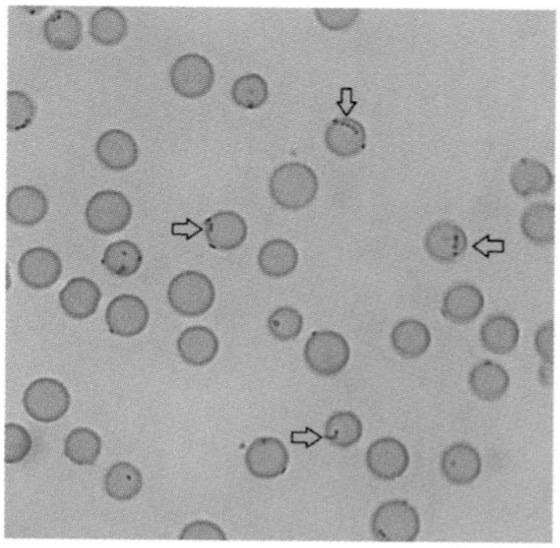 Figure 2.38 *Mycoplasma haemofelis* (arrows).

(*Continued*)

Table 2.8   (*Continued*)

Agent	Description	Image/examples
	Mycoplasma haemocanis (formerly *Haemobartonella canis*)	Dogs
	Mycoplasma haemofelis (formerly *Haemobartonella felis*)	Cats (also referred to as feline infectious anemia [FIA])
	Mycoplasma wenyonii (formerly *Eperythrozoon*)	Bovine
	Mycoplasma suis and *Mycoplasma parvum* (formerly *Eperythrozoon* spp.)	Pigs
	Mycoplasma haemolamae (formerly *Eperythrozoon*)	Llamas and alpacas
Microfilaria of *Dirofilaria immitis*	Larval stage of the nematode *Dirofilaria immitis* (canine heartworm)	

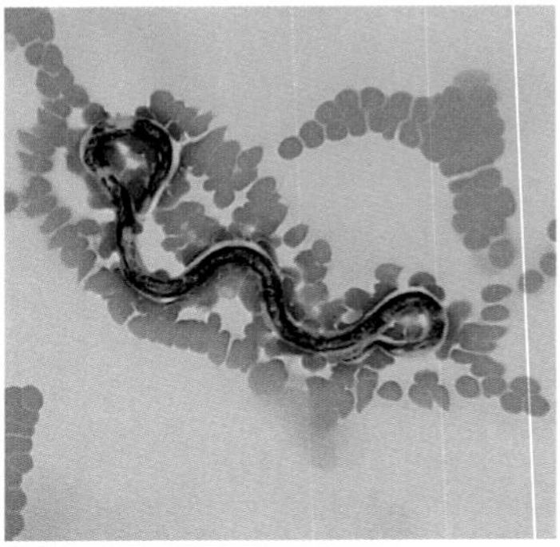

Figure 2.39 Microfilaria of *Dirofilaria immitis*.

Red cell arrangement

Table 2.9   Red cell arrangement

Arrangement	Description	Image/examples
Rouleaux	Erythrocytes are arranged in a chain formation. Associated with: Normal equines and some cats Inflammatory conditions and hyperglobulinemia	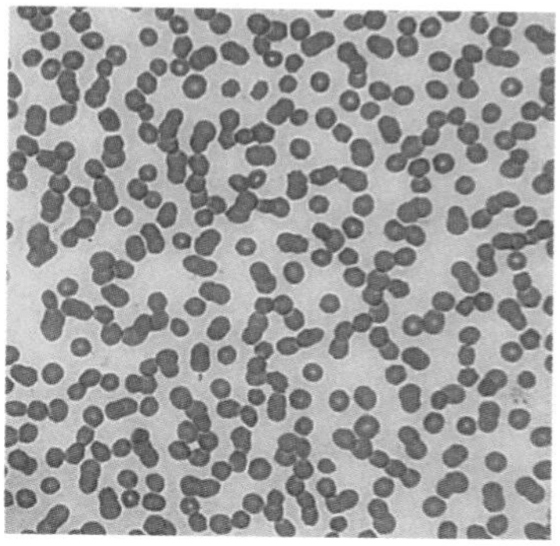 Figure 2.40 Rouleaux.
Agglutination	Erythrocytes are clumped together due to the binding of antibodies on the surfaces of the cells. Associated with IMHA	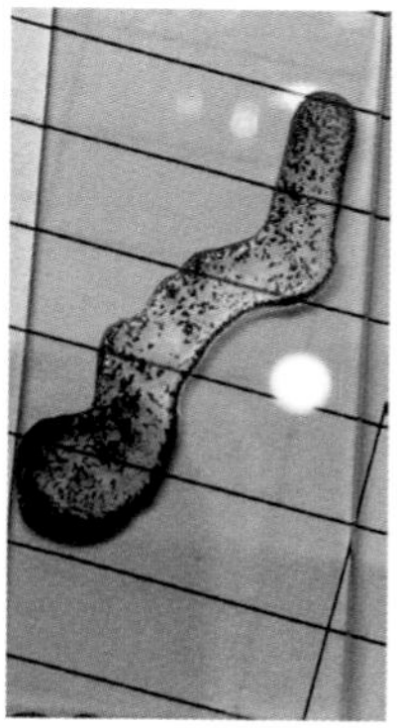 Figure 2.41 Macroscopic slide agglutination.

To differentiate rouleaux from agglutination, a saline dilution test should be performed.

Saline dilution test
In cases where rouleaux is heavy and indistinguishable from agglutination, the saline dilution test can be used to differentiate the two (Procedure 2.6).

Procedure 2.6   Saline dilution test to confirm agglutination

Materials
- EDTA blood sample
- 0.9% saline
- Microscope slide

- Coverslip
- Microscope

Procedure

(1) Perform a 1:5–1:10 dilution of EDTA blood to 0.9% saline. Add two drops of this dilution to a microscope slide.
(2) Place a coverslip over the drop.
(3) Examine using 400× magnification.
(4) Rouleaux will disperse using this technique, while agglutination will still remain present.

Artifacts

Table 2.10   Artifacts

Crenation	See *Echinocytes* Red cells possess small blunt spicules on the edge of the cell. Occurs as a result of prolonged exposure to EDTA anticoagulant or excessive EDTA anticoagulant which occurs with underfilling the blood tube.	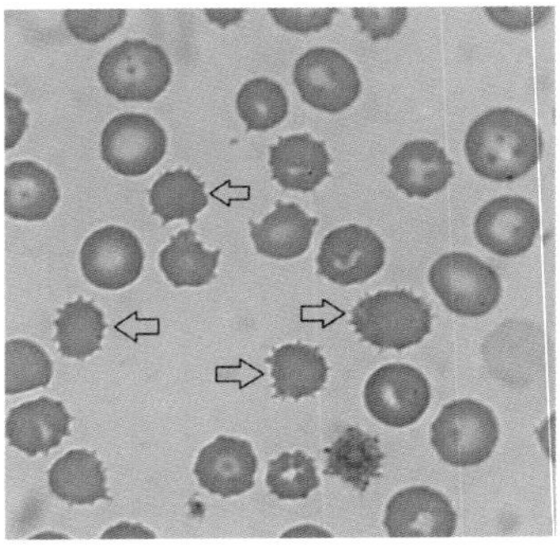 Figure 2.42 Crenation (arrows).
Stain precipitate	Aged stain will develop precipitate which may be transferred onto the smear. This can also occur with poor rinsing following the staining procedure. The stain precipitate will appear quite dark and on a different plane of focus than the cells. Often clumped and refractile (shiny looking)	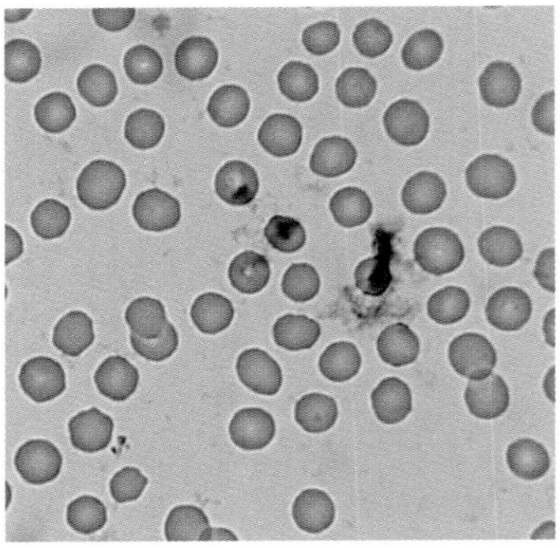 Figure 2.43 Stain precipitate seen as dark purple overlay of the cells.

Table 2.10 (*Continued*)

Water artifact	Gives a moth-eaten appearance to the erythrocytes. When focusing in and out, the artifact will appear refractile	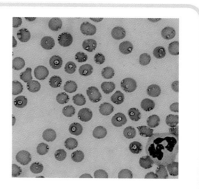 Figure 2.44 Water artifact. Note the refractile appearance of the cells.
Torocyte	Cells possess an increased central pallor, however the transition is abrupt, not gradual, as seen in hypochromic cells. Associated with incorrect smear spreading technique.	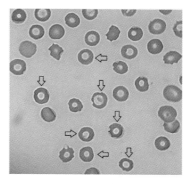 Figure 2.45 Torocytes (arrows).
Platelet overlap	On occasion, platelets can be laid on top of erythrocytes and may be confused with a parasite or inclusion.	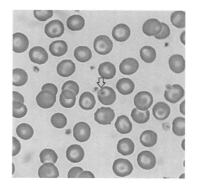 Figure 2.46 Platelet overlap (arrow).

The leukogram—WBC evaluation

Evaluating the leukogram includes counting the numbers of WBC, differentiating amongst the various types as well as reviewing their morphology. Mammalian species have 5 types of leukocytes (Table 2.11)

Table 2.11   Mammalian leukocytes

Neutrophils Eosinophils Basophils	Granulocytes
Lymphocytes Monocytes	Agranulocytes

WBC count

Procedure 2.7   WBC count

Materials
- Whole blood
- Isotonic dilution fluid with RBC lysing agent at 1:20 ratio (e.g., Leuko-TIC test kits, Bioanalytic GmbH)
- Improved Neubauer hemocytometer
- Coverslip (specific for a hemocytometer)
- Microscope with 10× lens objective
- Cell counter

Procedure
(1) Follow instructions of manufacturer of dilution medium to properly mix the blood sample.
(2) Place a clean coverslip on top of the hemocytometer.
(3) Flood one side of the hemocytometer counting chamber using capillary action.
(4) Using the 10× lens objective, count the WBCs within each the four big corner squares of the grid. (see Figure 2.47 and Figure 2.48).
(5) Repeat this count on the second side of the hemocytometer.
(6) Calculate totals for side 1 and side 2 of the hemocytometer grid and average.

Calculations
Calculations should be made using the average between Side 1 and Side 2.

QC
Side 1 and side 2 totals should be within 10% of each other before the average is taken.

$$\frac{average \times 50}{1000} = \underline{} \times 10^3 / \mu L$$

Sources of error
- Improper mixing of whole blood
- Improper filling of commercial dilution device or improper mixing prior to use

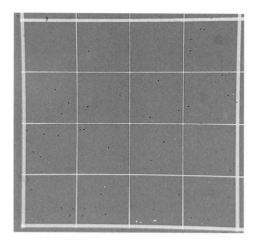

Figure 2.47 Microscopic view of hemocytometer grid with white blood cells (small dark pin point spots).

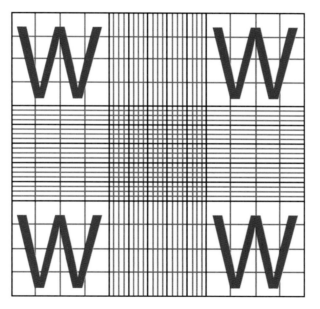

Figure 2.48 White blood cell counting area (W).

- Incomplete flooding or overfilling of the hemocytometer chamber
- Using a dirty hemocytometer, which can cause difficulty with differentiating between WBCs and debris.

WBC estimate

Performing a WBC estimate can be useful as a quick evaluation of a patient's leukocyte numbers if the materials required for a count are not available (Procedure 2.8). Estimates can also be done if an analyzer's WBC count is questionable or is flagged.

Procedure 2.8   WBC estimate

Materials
- Stained PBS
- Microscope with 40× lens objective
- Cell counter

Procedure
Examine a stained blood smear under 400× magnification.

(1) Count the number of leukocytes seen per field within the monolayer of the smear.
(2) Count 10 fields and calculate the average number of cells seen per field.

$$Average \times 1.5 = \underline{\hspace{2cm}} \times 10^3/\mu L$$

Sources of error
- Poorly made smear
- Counting in areas too thick or too thin (Figure 2.49).

WBC differential count

A WBC differential count gives information regarding the proportion and numbers of individual leukocytes in the patient's sample, including significant morphological changes. This can provide useful diagnostic information in cases of inflammation, infection, and antigenic responses (Procedure 2.9).

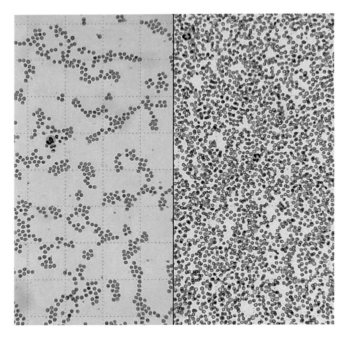

Figure 2.49   Areas of the smear that are too thin (left) and too thick (right).

Procedure 2.9   WBC differential count

Materials
- Stained PBS
- Microscope with 100× lens objective
- Cell counter

Procedure
(1) Scan the slide in a methodical grid pattern, in order not to cover the same area twice.

   Counts can be completed quickly under 400× magnification, but if you are also evaluating morphology, 1000× magnification should be used.

(2) Count a minimum of 100 WBCs. *(If the total WBC count is increased, 200 cells should be counted to maintain accuracy.)*

Calculations
Relative differential

$$\frac{\text{No. of cell type seen}}{100} = \underline{\quad\quad}\%$$

Absolute differential

$$\frac{\text{relative}\,(\%)}{100} \times \text{WBC count}\left(10^3/\mu L\right) = \underline{\quad\quad}\times 10^3/\mu L$$

Check your math:
- Relative counts of each cell type should add up to 100.
- Absolute counts of each cell type should add up to equal your WBC count.

It is important that examination and counts be performed within the monolayer area of the slide (Figure 2.50).

Corrected WBC count

Nucleated RBCs (NRBCs) can alter the accuracy of your WBC count. NRBCs (Figure 2.25) can be seen in cases of regenerative anemia and in some bone marrow disorders. This is because they are a nucleated cell (like a WBC) and are mistakenly recorded as such by the analyzer. This results in a falsely high WBC count. Performing a corrected white blood count adjusts your WBC count to account for these NRBCs (Procedure 2.10).

Procedure 2.10   Corrected WBC count

Materials
- Stained blood smear
- Microscope with 100× (oil immersion) lens objective
- Cell counter

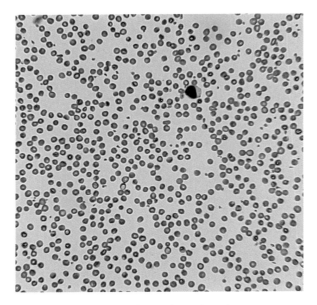

Figure 2.50 Microscopic view of the read area (monolayer).

Procedure

NRBCs are first noted during your slide evaluation, usually while performing a WBC differential count.

(1) During your 100-cell differential count, record the number of NRBCs seen.
(2) Do not include NRBCs as a part of your 100-cell WBC differential. Record them separately.

$$\frac{100}{100 + \text{no. of NRBCs}} \times \text{WBC count}\ \left(10^3/\mu L\right) \times 1000 = \underline{\quad\quad} \times 10^3/\mu L$$

Table 2.12 Leukocyte Morphology

WBC type	Description	Significance
Neutrophil (segmented neutrophil, mature neutrophil)	Segmented nucleus with coarsely clumped chromatin which stains dark purple. Cytoplasm is clear to pale blue. Granules are fine and may be difficult to visualize. Most commonly encountered leukocyte in dogs, cats and horses.	Phagocytosis of bacteria Circulate in the bloodstream for 10–15 hours before moving into the tissues. Neutrophilia may be seen in cases of infection, inflammation, stress or excitement. Neutropenia may be seen in instances of increased consumption by the tissues, sequestration of the cells or decreased production by the bone marrow.

Table 2.12 (*Continued*)

WBC type	Description	Significance
Band neutrophil	Immature stage of the neutrophil Predominantly in very low numbers in healthy animals Nucleus is band/rod/S shaped and lacks segmentation. Typically a darker cytoplasm Width of the nucleus is largely parallel with constriction being no more than 50% of the width. Band neutrophils should be counted separately from mature neutrophils. If the stage of development is difficult to determine due to borderline characteristics, then the cell should be counted as mature.	Increased band neutrophils are commonly seen in cases of inflammation. Increased band neutrophils can also be seen in leukemias. The presence of increased band neutrophils is termed "left shift."
Eosinophil	Similar in size to neutrophils. Numbers are low in normal animals. Nucleus is similar to that of neutrophils, however the number of segments varies by species but is typically less segmented than neutrophils. Occasionally a completed separated nucleus is seen (fully segmented). The cytoplasm is pale blue; however, it may be obscured by granules. The granules vary by species in their number, size, and color. Canine eosinophil granules vary in their size and stain a light pink. Greyhound (and other sighthounds) eosinophil granules are not visible and the cell will have a grey cytoplasm and appear to contain vacuoles. Equine eosinophil granules are quite large and fill the cell. Feline eosinophil granules are rod-shaped. Cattle and sheep eosinophils are round with intense pink staining	Eosinophilia is associated with a parasitic response and modulation of allergic inflammatory responses.
Basophil	Larger in size as compared to neutrophils. Rarely encountered in normal animals, however low numbers may be seen in healthy cattle and horses. Cytoplasm is grey-blue. The nucleus is segmented as other granulocytes and varies amongst species. The granules are purple staining; however they can vary in their intensity amongst species (pale lavender in canines and felines to dark purple in horses and ruminants)	The exact Function is not known; however, they are implicated in hypersensitivity reactions. Contain heparin and histamine.

(Continued)

Table 2.12 (*Continued*)

WBC type	Description	Significance
Lymphocyte	Most common cell seen in ruminants, second most common in dogs, cats and horses. In dogs, cats and horses, small lymphocytes are most commonly encountered (smaller than neutrophils). The nucleus is round with dense chromatin. The cytoplasm is scant and blue in color. In ruminants, intermediate to large-sized lymphocytes are seen (similar size to neutrophils). The chromatin is more loosely clumped and the cytoplasm is more abundant and light blue in color.	Composed of subpopulations which provide immunologic defense. These subpopulations cannot be definitively distinguished microscopically. Nucleated red blood cells (NRBCs) may be misidentified as small lymphocytes. Lymphocytosis is associated with an excitement response (fight/flight response), most commonly seen in cats. Lymphopenia is associated with a stress response, acute infection or lymph-rich effusions.
Monocyte	Seen in low numbers in healthy animals. Larger in size than neutrophils. They can be difficult to identify as they can vary greatly in their size and shape. The cytoplasm is grey-blue in color and may contain vacuoles and fine, light pink granules. The nucleus can vary in its shape from round, to kidney-shaped to band-shaped. The chromatin is loosely clumped and has a "lacy" appearance.	Monocytes migrate to the tissues where they become macrophages and phagocytose antigens and debris. Monocytosis is commonly seen in stress leukograms of dogs due to inflammation. Monocytes can be confused with lymphocytes, band neutrophils and metamyelocytes.

Normal species morphology

Table 2.13   Canine leukocytes

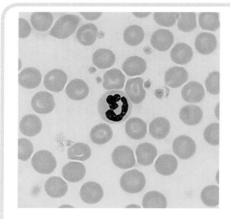

Figure 2.51   Canine neutrophil.

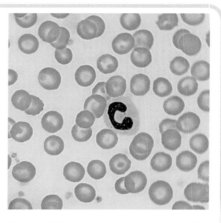

Figure 2.52   Canine band neutrophil.

Table 2.13   (*Continued*)

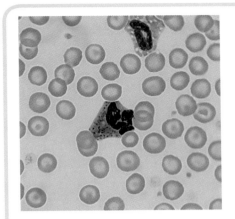

Figure 2.53   Canine basophil.

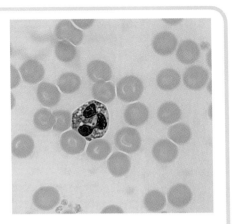

Figure 2.54   Canine eosinophil.

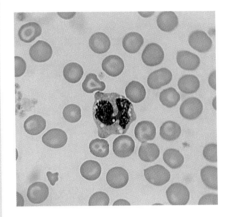

Figure 2.55   Canine monocyte.

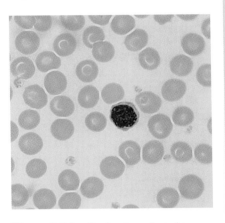

Figure 2.56   Canine lymphocyte.

Table 2.14   Feline leukocytes

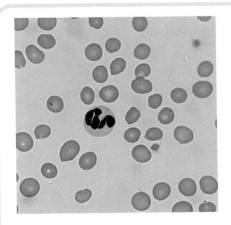

Figure 2.57   Feline neutrophil.

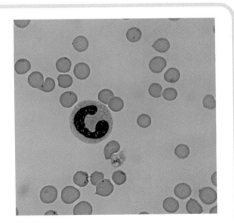

Figure 2.58   Feline band neutrophil.

(*Continued*)

Table 2.14 (*Continued*)

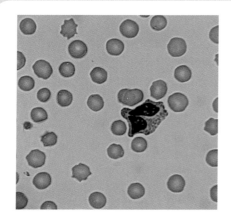

Figure 2.59 Feline basophil.

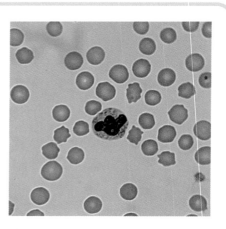

Figure 2.60 Feline eosinophil.

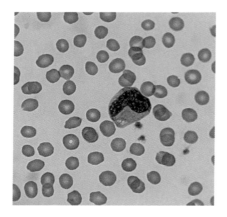

Figure 2.61 Feline monocyte.

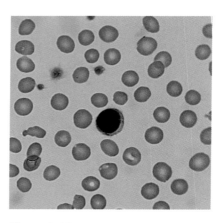

Figure 2.62 Feline lymphocyte.

Table 2.15 Equine leukocytes

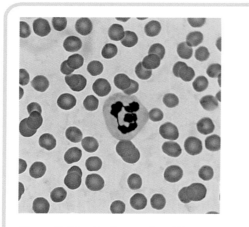

Figure 2.63 Equine neutrophil.

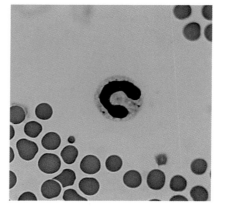

Figure 2.64 Equine band neutrophil.

Table 2.15   (Continued)

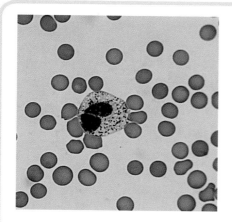

Figure 2.65   Equine basophil.

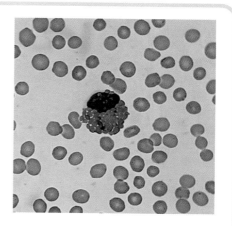

Figure 2.66   Equine eosinophil.

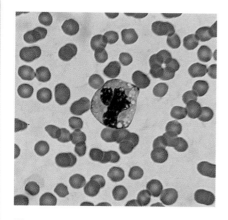

Figure 2.67   Equine monocyte.

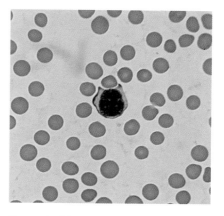

Figure 2.68   Equine lymphocyte.

Table 2.16   Bovine leukocytes

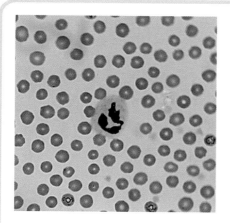

Figure 2.69   Bovine neutrophil.

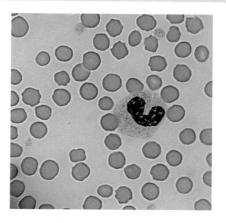

Figure 2.70   Bovine band neutrophil.

(Continued)

Table 2.16 (*Continued*)

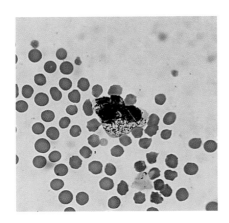

Figure 2.71   Bovine basophil.

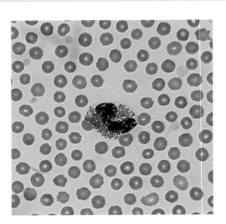

Figure 2.72   Bovine eosinophil.

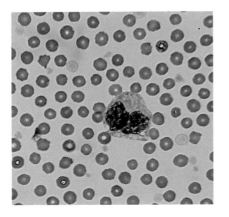

Figure 2.73   Bovine monocyte.

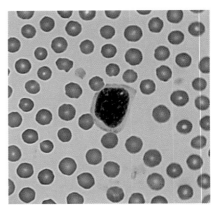

Figure 2.74   Bovine lymphocyte.

Table 2.17   Ovine leukocytes

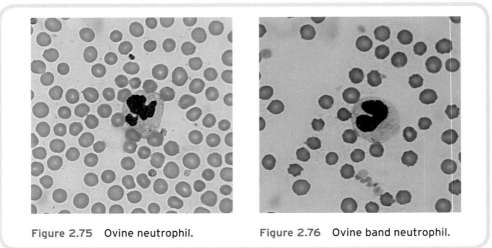

Figure 2.75   Ovine neutrophil.

Figure 2.76   Ovine band neutrophil.

Table 2.17 *(Continued)*

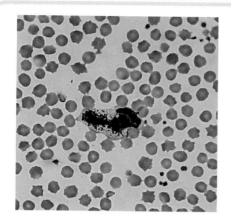

Figure 2.77   Ovine basophil.

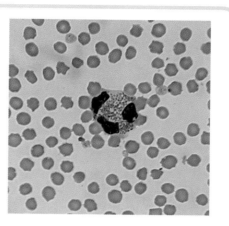

Figure 2.78   Ovine eosinophil.

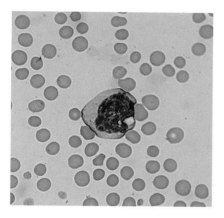

Figure 2.79   Ovine monocyte.

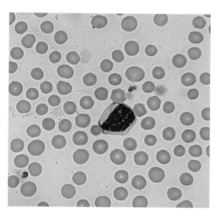

Figure 2.80   Ovine lymphocyte.

Abnormal and less commonly encountered leukocyte morphology descriptions

Table 2.18   Abnormal and less commonly encountered leukocyte morphology descriptions

Leukocyte	Description	Significance
Neutrophil hypersegmentation (Figure 2.81)	The nucleus of the cell possesses 5 or more segments or lobes	Natural maturing process of the neutrophil. Indicates an older neutrophil. Is seen as a result of retention in the blood stream and can be associated with corticosteroid treatment.

(Continued)

Table 2.18 (*Continued*)

Leukocyte	Description	Significance
Metamyelocyte (Figure 2.82)	The nucleus is bean-shaped with chromatin clumping that is less than a band. The cytoplasm is a deeper blue.	An immature neutrophil, one stage younger than a band neutrophil. Rarely encountered. Associated with an inflammatory leukogram. Can be misidentified as a monocyte.
Toxic neutrophil (Figure 2.83)	Neutrophils possess several possible morphologies • Döhle bodies: pale blue inclusions in the cytoplasm (aggregates of endoplasmic reticulum) • Cytoplasmic basophilia: increased blue coloring to the cytoplasm • Vacuoles: gives the neutrophils a "foamy" appearance • Toxic granulation: pink-purple-staining granules	Toxic changes are due to accelerated neutrophil production in the bone marrow. This acceleration is typically in response to inflammation (infectious or noninfectious). Healthy cats can have low numbers of Döhle bodies present.
Pelger-Huet anomaly	Mature neutrophils which are hyposegmented. Nuclear chromatin is condensed, as it is in normal, mature neutrophils. Function is normal. Also referred to as a "false left shift"	Genetic disorder seen in some dog breeds such as Australian Shepherds. Important not to misidentify these cells as band neutrophils.
Barr body (Figure 2.84)	A "drumstick"-looking appendage on the nucleus.	Seen on the neutrophil nuclei of female animals.
Granular lymphocytes (Figure 2.85)	Lymphocytes contain small red granules.	Small numbers are seen in normal animals. Increased numbers are associated with reactive conditions (ie: *Ehrlichia canis* infections)
Reactive lymphocytes (Figure 2.86)	The nucleus contains clumped chromatin. May appear slightly larger with darker, more abundant cytoplasm. Nucleoli are often visible within the nucleus. A perinuclear clear zone is visible.	Associated with an antigenic response. More commonly seen in young animals which have recently been vaccinated. May be misidentified as immature blast cells.

Table 2.19   Abnormal and less commonly encountered leukocyte morphology images

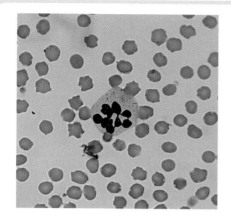

Figure 2.81   Neutrophil hypersegmentation.

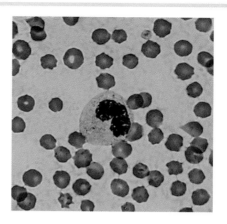

Figure 2.82   Metamyelocyte.

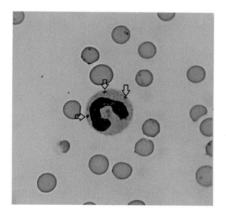

Figure 2.83 Toxic neutrophil with Döhle bodies (arrows).

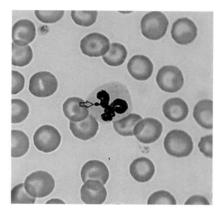

Figure 2.84   Barr body (arrow).

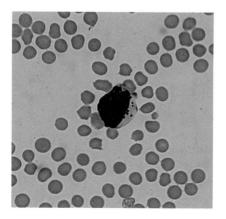

Figure 2.85   Granular lymphocyte.

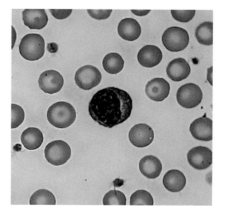

Figure 2.86 Reactive lymphocyte. (Note the perinuclear clear zone adjacent to the nucleus)

Commonly encountered leukograms

Inflammatory leukogram

During an inflammatory occurrence, cytokines are released and stimulate the bone marrow to release stored neutrophils as well as band (immature) neutrophils. Causes of inflammation vary greatly and can include infectious agents, noninfectious events, and autoimmune-mediated conditions, among others. The following changes can be seen.

(1) Neutrophilia: increased numbers of segmented neutrophils
(2) Left shift: increased numbers of band (immature) neutrophils

Other possible changes in the leukogram
(1) Toxic change (Table 2.18)
(2) Monocytosis (more commonly noted when the inflammation in chronic)

Regenerative left shift
A regenerative left shift is noted when neutrophilia is present, along with an increase in band neutrophils. The number of mature (segmented) neutrophils exceeds the number of band (immature) neutrophils.

Degenerative left shift
A degenerative left shift is noted when the neutrophil numbers are within normal limits or decreased (neutropenia). An increase of band neutrophils is also noted. The number of band (immature) neutrophils exceeds the number of mature (segmented) neutrophils. Immature neutrophils can also represent metamyelocytes, which may be seen in severe cases when the demand is high.

Stress leukogram

A stress leukogram is the result of the influence of corticosteroids, either endogenous (e.g., cortisol) or exogenous (e.g., dexamethasone and prednisone). This causes a mature neutrophilia due to increased levels of retention of the neutrophils within the circulation. Hypersegmentation of the neutrophils may also be observed (Table 2.18). Another consistent change is lymphopenia. Monocytosis may be observed; however, it is seen most consistently in dogs with a stress leukogram. A stress leukogram may also be seen concurrently with an inflammatory response, in which case, immature neutrophils will also be noted.

Physiological (excitement) leukogram

A physiologic, or excitement, response is due to epinephrine response and may also be referred to as the "fight or flight" response. The effects of epinephrine cause an increase of blood flow through the microcirculation, resulting in the flushing of mature neutrophils into circulation. This causes mature neutrophilia as well as lymphocytosis. There is no increase in band neutrophils. The physiological response is the most pronounced in cats.

The thrombogram—platelet evaluation

Platelet count

Procedure 2.11 Platelet count

Materials
- Whole blood
- Isotonic dilution fluid to preserve platelets at a 1:20 ratio (e.g. Thrombo-TIC test kit, Bioanalytic GmbH)
- Improved Neubauer hemocytometer
- Coverslip
- Microscope with 40× lens objective
- Cell counter

Procedure
(1) Follow instructions of manufacturer of dilution medium to properly mix the blood sample.
(2) Place a clean coverslip on top of the hemocytometer.
(3) Flood one side of the hemocytometer counting chamber using capillary action.
(4) Count the platelets within 25 group squares (Figure 2.87).
(5) Repeat this count on the second side of the hemocytometer. Counts should not be done if platelet clumping is seen. If clumping is noted, repeat the dilution or collect a new blood sample if clumping persists.
(6) Calculate totals for side 1 and side 2 of the hemocytometer grid and average.

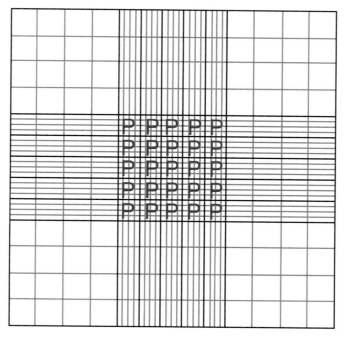

Figure 2.87   Platelet counting area (P).

Calculations
Calculations should be made using the average between side 1 and side 2.

QC
Side 1 and side 2 totals should be within 10% of each other before the average is taken.

$$average = \underline{\hspace{1cm}} \times 10^3/\mu L$$

Sources of error
- Improper mixing of whole blood
- Improper filling of commercial dilution device or improper mixing prior to use
- Incomplete flooding or overfilling of the hemocytometer chamber
- Using a dirty hemocytometer, which can cause difficulty with differentiating between platelets and debris
- Platelet clumping present due to collection and/or handling of the blood sample

Platelet estimate

Performing a platelet estimate is a quick and simple way to verify adequate platelet numbers in a patient's sample (Procedure 2.12). It is also useful when errors and flags arise during automated analysis of blood. Depending upon the analyzer, macroplatelets, which are large platelets (see Figure 2.88), and platelet clumping can cause false readings.

Procedure 2.12 Platelet estimate

Materials
- Stained PBS
- Microscope with 100× lens objective
- Cell counter

Procedure
(1) First, scan the edges of the smear under low power for platelet clumps.
(2) Because clumps are larger than individual cells, they will be pushed to the outer edges of the smear.

> *Tip*: **Platelet clumping is a common occurrence following the collection of blood from cats and horses. To avoid clumping, make a blood smear using fresh blood immediately following collection, before any anticoagulant is added. If no clumping is seen, proceed with the estimate.**

(3) Examine a stained blood smear under 1000× magnification.
(4) Count the number of platelets seen per field within the monolayer of the smear.
(5) Count 10 fields and calculate the average number of cells seen per field.

$$average \times 20 = \underline{\hspace{1cm}} \times 10^3/\mu L$$

Platelet estimates may also be reported as "adequate"; however, that is subjective. For the average mammal, 6–10 platelets per field (1000× magnification) is considered adequate.

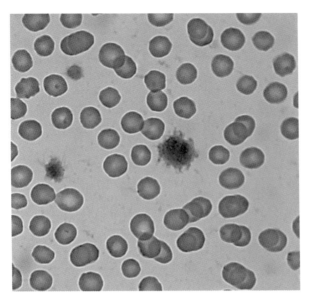

Figure 2.88   Typical platelet (left) compared to a macroplatelet (right).

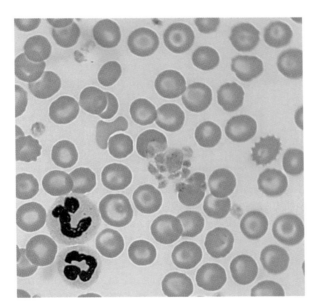

Figure 2.89   Platelet clumping.

Sources of error
- Poorly made smear
- Counting in areas too thick or too thin
- Platelet clumping present (Figure 2.89).

Platelet morphology

Normal morphology

Platelets are cytoplasmic fragments which arise from the megakaryocyte cell in the bone marrow. They are anuclear with a pale blue cytoplasm and contain small, pink granules. Activated platelets possess spiny extensions on their surface. The size of platelets varies greatly among species and within the sample itself. Feline samples typically have a large variation in platelet sizes.

Platelet clumping

Once activated, platelets develop extensions and begin to aggregate. This can be seen on a blood film and is noted as platelet clumping. A common cause of platelet clumping is delayed exposure of the blood sample to an anticoagulant during collection. Cats have highly reactive platelets which clump readily during collection.

Mean platelet volume

Mean platelet volume (MPV) is a calculated value generated by analyzers which represents the size of the average platelet in the sample. An increased MPV suggests larger-than-normal platelets (on average) within the sample. Platelet clumping can artificially increase the MPV; therefore, a blood film should be evaluated to rule out the presence of clumps.

Plateletcrit

Expressed as a percentage, the plateletcrit (PCT) is a value generated by automated analyzers which represents the average platelet mass. The calculation incorporates the MPV as well as the platelet count; therefore, erroneous results present in either of these values due to poor sample quality (e.g., platelet clumping) will also affect the PCT.

Point-of-care coagulation testing

Hemostasis consists of primary hemostasis (platelet component) and secondary hemostasis (actions of coagulation factors). Coagulation testing is a broad topic which includes a number of testing procedures to evaluate each of these components.

Primary hemostasis testing

Primary hemostasis testing includes evaluating platelet numbers by performing a platelet count or platelet estimate. It also includes assessing platelet function by performing a buccal mucosal bleeding time (BMBT) test.

Buccal mucosal bleeding time (BMBT) test

Procedure 2.13   BMBT test

Materials
- Patient sedation/anesthesia
- Gauze to secure the upper lip

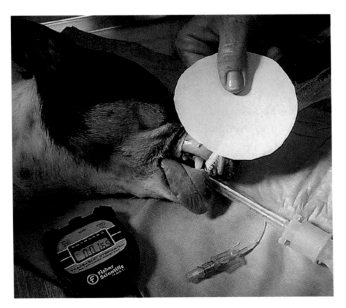

Figure 2.90 Buccal mucosal bleeding time test. (From Sirois M, *Principles and Practice of Veterinary Technology*, 4th ed. Saunders-Elsevier, St. Louis, MO, 2017). *Source:* From Margi Sirois, (2017), ELSEVIER.

- Lancet
- Stopwatch
- Filter paper/gauze

Procedure
(1) Anesthetize/sedate the patient and place in lateral recumbency.
(2) Fold the upper lip of the patient up and secure with gauze.
(3) Create a small incision using a spring-loaded lancet in the mucosa of the lip above the premolars. Different lancets vary from 2.5 to 6 mm long by 0.5 to 1 mm deep. The size lancet used based on patient size should be standardized in the clinic.
(4) Start the timer.
(5) Wick away the blood from the incision site with filter paper, but do not touch the incision site (Figure 2.90).
(6) Continue to remove the blood at 5-second intervals.
(7) Record the time when the blood is no longer flowing and being absorbed into the filter paper.

Reference interval
1-5 minutes

Sources of error
There are many variables that can be introduced into this testing procedure. Examples include the depth of the cut, how the upper lip is secured, and patient management. Variables should be minimized as much as possible, and procedures standardized.

Secondary hemostasis testing

To assess the coagulation factors included in the extrinsic, intrinsic, and common coagulation pathways, point-of-care coagulation analyzers are available.

Activated coagulation time—manual method

The activated coagulation time (ACT) test is used to assess the coagulation factors of the intrinsic and common pathways. (Procedure 2.14)

Prothrombin time and activated partial thromboplastin time

Prothrombin time (PT), also called one-stage prothrombin time (OSPT), assesses the extrinsic and the common pathways, while activated partial PT (aPTT) is used to assess the factors of the intrinsic and common pathways. For both procedures, blood is collected in a citrate anticoagulant tube. Samples are run on point-of-care analyzers to assess secondary hemostasis.

Fibrinogen testing

Fibrinogen concentration can be measured using manually and automated methods. The manual heat precipitation method is the least accurate method but does not require specialized equipment. (Procedure 2.15)

Procedure 2.14   ACT—manual method
Materials
- Fresh venous blood
- Blood collection tube containing diatomaceous earth
- Stopwatch
- Incubator or warm water bath to maintain temperature
- Thermometer

Procedure
(1) Draw 2 mL of venous blood into a prewarmed tube (37°C) containing diatomaceous earth.
(2) Begin timing immediately.
(3) Invert the tube several times.
(4) Continue to keep the tube at 37°C using an incubator or warm water bath.
(5) After 1 minute, continue to check for clot formation every 5–10 seconds.
(6) Stop the time when a clot forms.

Reference intervals
Dogs: 79 ± 7.1 seconds
Horses: 163 ± 18 seconds
Cows: 145 ± 18 seconds

Alternatively, automated ACT testing can be assessed with the use of point-of-care coagulation analyzers.

Procedure 2.15 Manual fibrinogen testing (heat precipitation method)

Materials
- EDTA blood
- Microhematocrit tubes
- Tube sealant
- Centrifuge
- Incubator or warm water bath
- Refractometer

Procedure
(1) Prepare 2 microhematocrit tubes as would be done for a PCV. Make a counter-balance PCV tube.
(2) Centrifuge one tube, then using a refractometer measure the total solids of the tube.
(3) Incubate the second tube at 58°C for 3 minutes.
(4) Centrifuge the second tube.
(5) Measure the total solids of the second tube.

Fibrinogen estimate is the difference between the two readings.

Automated hematology

In-house automated hematology is a useful tool for the veterinary technologist. It allows the technologist to process many samples quickly and efficiently. Hematology analyzers, if maintained correctly, also have a high level of accuracy and precision, making them a reliable tool for patient diagnosis.

As technology continues to advance, it is important to understand how the technologist's role evolves as well. A technologist is more than just an operator. He or she needs to be able to ensure that the results provided are correct and complete before reporting them to the veterinarian. To accomplish this, a knowledge of the technology, capability, and limitations of the analyzer being utilized is very important.

Understanding the limitations or error messages of an analyzer can guide the technologist to perform a manual blood film for review. Evaluating a blood film in tandem with the analyzer can provide supportive information regarding morphology, hemoparasites, and platelet clumping and help to confirm the accuracy of the analyzer results.

Evaluating a blood film to verify automated results

Evaluating a blood film should not be a tedious task. Its purposes are to confirm the analyzer's values, to investigate flags or error messages, and to review characteristics which the analyzer is unable to provide (e.g., cell morphologies).

100× magnification review
- Examine the feathered edge for cell clumping.
- Scan the monolayer of the film to review the cell density and RBC arrangement.

400× magnification review
- Validate the WBC differential and possibility of reticulocytosis if necessary (polychromatic RBCs).
- Examine RBC, WBC, and platelet morphologies.

1000× magnification review
- Validate the platelet count by counting the average number of platelets per field.

Cytograms

Automated analyzers generate a cytogram, which is a graphic representation of cell populations and distributions. The type of cytogram generated depends on the type of analyzer. Histograms and dot plots are examples of common cytograms.

Chapter 3
Chemistry and Serology

Chemistry

To evaluate the function of most body systems, clinical chemistries, enzymes, and compounds are analyzed to give a picture of how well the body is working. The majority of chemical tests will require either a serum or plasma sample (Procedures 3.1 and 3.2). Some analyzers are able to process anticoagulated whole blood by automatically extracting the plasma without the need for centrifugation.

Serum and plasma are both the fluid portion of whole blood and include constituents such as, but not limited to, proteins, hormones, enzymes, antibodies, and lipids. Plasma contains the protein fibrinogen, while serum does not. When blood is allowed to clot, the fibrinogen is converted to fibrin and included in the clot. To obtain a plasma sample, an anticoagulant must be used to prevent clotting. Normal plasma and serum are pale yellow and clear. Horses normally have a brighter yellow coloration to both.

Sample processing and types

Procedure 3.1   Plasma sample preparation

- Collect a blood sample using the appropriate anticoagulant tube. Care should be taken to avoid clotting during collection. Mix well by gently inverting.
- Centrifuge the sample at 2000 to 3000 rpm for 10 minutes.
- Remove the plasma, being careful not to disturb the cell layer.
- Transfer the plasma to a secondary labeled tube.
- Process immediately or refrigerate or freeze if desired.

Procedure 3.2   Serum sample preparation

- Collect a blood sample using a tube which contains no anticoagulant.
- Allow the blood to fully clot at room temperature. This could take 20 to 30 minutes.
- Separate the clot from the wall of the tube by carefully running a wooden applicator stick between the wall and the clot. If done improperly, there is a risk of creating artifactual hemolysis.

Veterinary Technician's Handbook of Laboratory Procedures, Second Edition. Brianne Bellwood and Melissa Andrasik-Catton.
© 2023 John Wiley & Sons, Inc. Published 2023 by John Wiley & Sons, Inc.
Companion website: www.wiley.com/go/bellwoodhandbook2

- Centrifuge the sample at 2000 to 3000 rpm for 10 minutes.
- Remove the serum, being careful not to disturb the cell layer (especially if a serum separator tube was not used).
- Transfer the serum to a secondary labeled tube.
- Process immediately or refrigerate or freeze if desired.

Sample quality concerns

Chemistry testing accuracy can be affected by a poor-quality sample, which could be a result of collection or handling or related to the patient's physiological status (Table 3.1). Three major quality concerns are hemolysis (Figure 3.1), lipemia and icterus. Care should be taken to avoid any human errors which could result in these sample quality concerns. If possible, patient preparation should be considered to avoid sample issues (e.g., fasting). The degree of interference from hemolysis, lipemia, or icterus with clinical chemistries and other tests is related to the intensity of each abnormality.

Table 3.1 Sample quality

Feature	Cause	Appearance	Affects
Hemolysis	Rupturing of RBCs Caused by: Forcing the blood through a small-gauge needle Shaking the blood vigorously Aged blood sample Freezing the sample Seen in patients with hemolytic anemia	Orange to red tinge to plasma or serum Degree of color change is related to the level of hemolysis in the sample	• Potassium • AST • Phosphate • CK • GGT • ALP Can affect RBC indices
Lipemia	Increased lipids in the plasma/serum Caused by: Sampling shortly after the animal has eaten a meal Can be disease related (e.g. canine pancreatitis)	Plasma/serum is opaque and white	• Sodium • Chloride • Magnesium • Triglyceride • Lipase Can interfere with bile acid and phenobarbital levels
Icterus	Increased levels of bilirubin in the plasma/serum Caused by: Hemolytic anemia Liver dysfunction	Plasma/serum displays an increased yellow coloring Most interference seen with very high levels of pigmentation	• Creatinine • Cholesterol • GGT

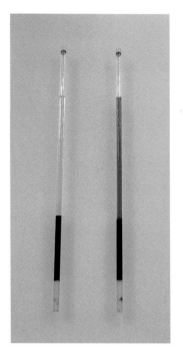

Figure 3.1   Normal plasma appearance (left) and hemolyzed plasma (right) in PCV tubes.

Blood collection tubes

A number of different blood collection tubes are available for the collection and processing of blood (Table 3.2 and Figure 3.2). Blood tubes contain the appropriate amount of anticoagulant for the capacity of the tube. It is important to maintain the intended anticoagulant:blood ratio to ensure a good quality sample.

Table 3.2   Common blood collection tubes

Blood tube	Tube top color	Contents	Uses
Red top (RTT)	Red	None	Serum samples
Serum separator (SST)	Gold or striped red top (tiger top)	Separator gel	Serum samples
Heparin (GTT)	Green	Heparin (lithium or sodium)	Plasma chemistry testing
Plasma separator (PST)	Green	Heparin; separator gel	Plasma chemistry testing
EDTA (LTT)	Purple (lavender)	K2 EDTA (or K3 EDTA)	Hematology
Citrate (BTT)	Blue	Sodium citrate	Coagulation testing

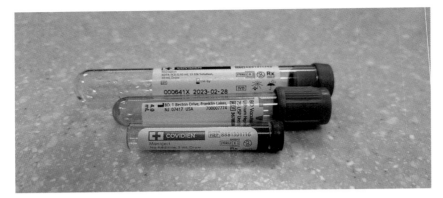

Figure 3.2 Various common blood collection tubes. EDTA, heparin, and red top (top to bottom).

Desired order of draw

Table 3.3 Order of draw

Order	Blood tube
1st	Sodium citrate (BTT)
2nd	Serum tubes (RTT or SST)
3rd	Heparin tubes (GTT, PST)
4th	EDTA (LTT)

Summary of chemistry tests

Table 3.4 Common chemistry tests

Liver injury	**Gastrointestinal system**
Aspartate aminotransferase (AST)	Amylase (AMY)
Alanine aminotransferase (ALP)	Lipase (LIP)
Liver function	Trypsin-like immunoreactivity (TLI)
Total bilirubin (TBIL)	**Endocrine function (parathyroid)**
Direct bilirubin	Parathyroid hormone (PTH)
Indirect bilirubin	Calcium (Ca^+)
Bile acids (BA)	Phosphorus (P^-)
Cholesterol (CHOL)	**Endocrine function (thyroid)**
Glucose (GLU)	Thyroid stimulating hormone (TSH)
Total protein (TP)	Thyroxine (total T4)
Albumin (ALB)	Free T4
Globulin (GLOB)	Cholesterol (CHOL)
Fibrinogen	Total protein (TP)
Cholestasis	**Endocrine function (adrenal)**
Alkaline phosphatase (ALP)	Glucose (GLU)
γ-Glutamyltransferase (GGT)	Cortisol
Total bilirubin (TBIL)	Cholesterol (CHOL)
Direct bilirubin	Alkaline phosphatase (ALP)
Indirect bilirubin	Sodium (Na^+)
	Potassium (K^+)

Table 3.4 *(Continued)*

Renal function	Electrolytes and minerals
Creatinine (CREA)	Bicarbonate (HCO$_3^-$)
Blood urea nitrogen (BUN)	Calcium (Ca$^+$)
Symmetric dimethylarginine (SDMA)	Chloride (Cl$^-$)
Pancreatic (endocrine)	Magnesium (Mg$^+$)
Glucose (GLU)	Phosphorus (P$^-$)
Pancreatic (exocrine)	Potassium (K$^+$)
Amylase (AMY)	Sodium (Na$^+$)
Lipase (LIP)	**Muscle damage**
Trypsin-like immunoreactivity (TLI)	Creatine kinase (CK)
Species-specific pancreatic lipase (cPLI = dogs; fPLI = cats)	Aspartate aminotransferase (AST)
	Lactate dehydrogenase (LD)

This represents common tests and is not intended to be an exhaustive list of possible chemistries.

Serology

Serologic testing involves the detection of specific antigens or antibodies in the patient sample. Typically, a serum or plasma sample is required; however, anticoagulated whole blood may also be suitable. There are several in-house kits available to perform these diagnostic tests. When using these tests, it is important to read the manufacturer's recommendations for sample type and sample quality considerations.

Common in-house serological tests

ELISA

The enzyme-linked immunosorbent assay (ELISA) is a common in-house test kit that has been tailored to detect a variety of components, such as viruses, bacteria, hormones, and parasites (Figure 3.3). ELISA testing relies on the binding of specific antigens and antibodies and, with an added color change enzymatic reaction, will produce a visible positive result. These tests can detect either the antigen or the antibody in a patient sample.

Competitive ELISA (CELISA) uses the same principles as the ELISA; however; in this case, the antigens in the patient sample must compete for antibodies with the antigens within the test kit to produce a color reaction.

Latex agglutination

The latex agglutination test uses latex particles coated in antigen, which bind with antibodies within the patient sample (if present). An antigen-antibody complex is formed and is confirmed by the presence of clumping (agglutination) (Figure 3.4).

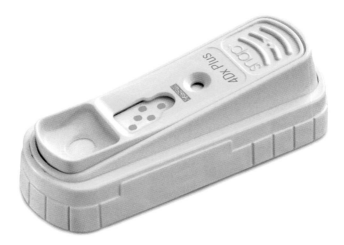

Figure 3.3 ELISA. A positive reaction is confirmed with a color change dot. (Photo of the IDEXX SNAP® 4Dx® Plus test provided courtesy of IDEXX Laboratories, Inc.)

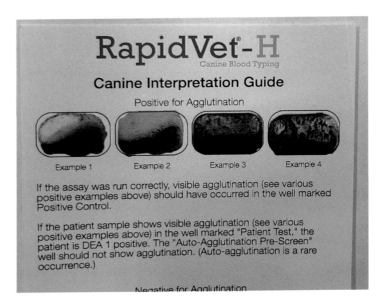

Figure 3.4 Latex agglutination test. A positive reaction is seen as clumping, whereas in a negative reaction, the sample remains smooth.

Rapid immunomigration

Also known as lateral flow tests, rapid immunomigration (RIM) tests also rely on antigen-antibody complexes and incorporate colloidal gold particles and color change reagents, which accumulate and produce a color change in a positive test.

Additional testing

Additional testing can be performed at reference labs and may include other testing principles such as immunodiffusion, antibody titers, fluorescent antibody testing,

DNA/RNA analysis, and polymerase chain reactions (PCR). These are specialized tests and do not lend themselves to being performed in-house.

Testing accuracy

Test kits are assessed for sensitivity and specificity. The sensitivity of a test demonstrates the ability to detect true positives. A test with high sensitivity will be able to detect low levels of antigens in the patient's sample. A test with low sensitivity will produce false negatives. The specificity of a test demonstrates the ability to detect and react with the intended antigen in the sample. The lower the specificity of a test, the higher the likelihood it will react with the incorrect antigen and produce a false positive.

Test kits will incorporate a positive control and potentially a negative control as well. The positive control ensures that the test and its components are working properly and provides assurance that the results can be accepted. If a test's positive control does not give the correct result, the results should be discarded, and the cause of the error should be investigated.

Chapter 4
Urinalysis

Conducting a thorough urinalysis involves observation of the physical attributes, chemical properties, and microscopic characteristics of an animal's urine sample, which can provide invaluable information about the current health status of the patient. The proficiency and experience of the person performing the analysis can dramatically affect the results reported, especially with sedimentation evaluation. It is encouraged, if unexpected results are obtained, that a second person conduct the analysis.

Sample collection and handling

Urine sample collection and handling are important preanalytic variables which affect the quality of the results produced from the analysis. The choice of collection method should consider the desired analysis (e.g., culture and sensitivity) as well as the practicality given the current situation and patient (Table 4.1). It is important to note the method of collection, the timing of collection, and the preservation method used (if any) when performing a urinalysis.

Urine should be collected and stored in sterile collection containers (Figure 4.1). A plain, glass red-top blood collection tube can also be used to store urine; plastic tubes are not recommended, as they contain clot activators which will introduce microscopic artifacts into the sample.

Voided sample

Samples collected through natural micturition is the least invasive method of collection. Obtaining the sample by free catch, bladder expression, tabletop or floor collection, or litter box can be utilized; however, contamination should be expected. Although steps can be taken to minimize this, none of these collection methods are suitable for culture and sensitivity testing.

Free-catch sample collection best practices
- Clean the vulva or prepuce prior to collection.
- Use a sterile specimen container for collection whenever possible.

Veterinary Technician's Handbook of Laboratory Procedures, Second Edition. Brianne Bellwood and Melissa Andrasik-Catton.
© 2023 John Wiley & Sons, Inc. Published 2023 by John Wiley & Sons, Inc.
Companion website: www.wiley.com/go/bellwoodhandbook2

Table 4.1 Urine collection methods

Method	Advantages	Disadvantages
Voided	• Noninvasive • Owners can perform at home	• High level of contamination
Bladder expression	• Urine collected at time it is needed	• High level of contamination • Risk of damage to bladder • Risk of reflux of urine into the kidneys • Patient resistant to procedure
Catheterization	• Minimized contamination relative to the voided method • Useful if bladder is not palpable for expression	• More invasive • May require sedation • Requires higher level of skill • May introduce bacteria into bladder
Cystocentesis	• Sterile technique (suitable for culture)	• More invasive • Requires higher level of skill • Likely to cause mild hematuria

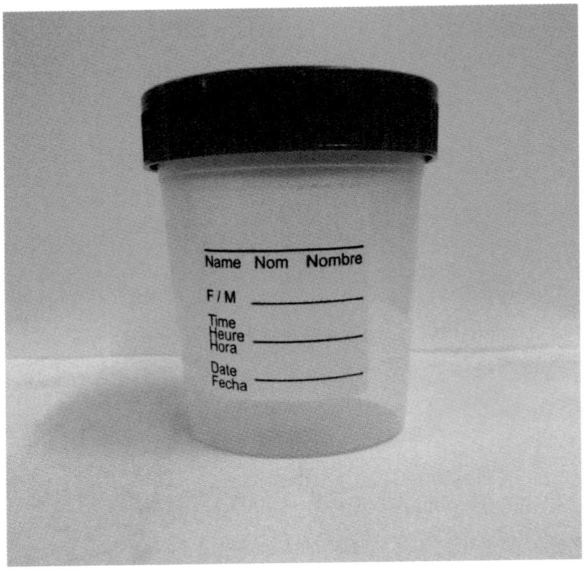

Figure 4.1 Urine collection container.

- Collect a midstream sample (avoid the first portion of the urine stream as it will be the most heavily contaminated with bacteria and debris).
- Using a collection cup with a long handle can be useful for male dogs. For female dogs, using a shallow collection container such as a pie plate allows better access.

Tabletop or floor collection best practices
- The surface is often highly contaminated with bacteria, which should be taken into account when analyzing the urine.
- If the table has been recently disinfected, it is important to be aware that many disinfectants can cause false results in the chemical examination of urine.

Litter box best practices
- The litter box should be clean. Lining the box with a trash bag can help minimize contamination.
- Use nonabsorbent litter such as packing peanuts or glass beads.
- Remove the urine immediately and transfer to a storage container.

Bladder expression best practices
- This technique should be used with caution, as it can result in the reflux of urine into the ureters and up to the kidneys.
- A forceful technique can result in trauma to the bladder, causing iatrogenic hematuria.
- Bladder expression should never be performed in patients with suspected urinary blockages.

Catheterization

Catheterization to obtain a urine sample is more invasive than the voided method and requires more skill. Sterile technique is essential to avoid introducing bacteria into the patient's urinary tract. Sedation may be required, especially in cats and female dogs.

Best practices for sample integrity
- Follow appropriate collection protocol given the sex and species of the patient.
- Use sterile equipment.
- Cleanse the external genitalia prior to collection.
- Discard the first portion of collected urine as it will contain nondiagnostic bacteria, cells, and debris from the distal urethra.
- Contamination of the sample by the lubricant used during catheterization is possible.

Cystocentesis

Cystocentesis is the method of choice for bacterial culture of a urine sample. The bladder can be located using palpation or with ultrasound guidance.

Best practices for sample integrity
- Follow appropriate collection protocol.
- Use sterile equipment.
- Mild hematuria is commonly seen as a side effect to this procedure.

Timing of sample collection

Depending on the purpose of the urinalysis, the timing of collection may be of importance. A first morning sample consists of urine which has been stored in the bladder for an extended period and is the most concentrated. This retention could cause the degradation of some elements (e.g., cellular elements and casts) or the formation/proliferation of others (e.g., crystals). A postprandial urine sample will be reflective of the diet, while a sample taken after fasting will be free of any diet-related metabolites. These factors should be considered when performing a urinalysis.

Sample preservation

Urine should be analyzed within 30 minutes of collection; delay in analysis can result in many in vitro changes (Table 4.2). Bacterial growth can decrease glucose and increase the pH. This change in pH can affect cellular and crystal elements of urine as well as the degeneration of casts.

Refrigeration

Refrigeration of urine is the most common method of extending the analysis window of urine for an additional 2 to 12 hours. While it will delay the proliferation of bacteria, it can also cause unwanted changes. Cold urine will read a higher specific gravity (SG) and precipitate amorphous crystals and also has the potential to inhibit the enzymatic reactions on the chemistry strips.

To avoid these negative consequences, refrigerated urine should be allowed to warm to room temperature prior to testing but not set on a counter, in light, for extended periods.

Freezing

Freezing is another method of preserving urine. While it is unsuitable for cellular elements, it is an option for preserving the chemical components of urine.

Table 4.2 In vitro changes in unpreserved urine

Substance	Change
Bacteria	Levels increase as bacteria proliferate
Bilirubin	Exposure to light will cause a decrease
Color	Darkens
Crystals	Increase or decrease depending on type. Occurs as a result of fluctuating pH
Erythrocytes	Dilute urine can cause hemolysis.
Glucose	Decreases as cells and bacteria metabolize the glucose for energy
Ketones	Decrease as acetone is volatile
Odor	Becomes stronger as bacteria produce more ammonia
pH	Typically becomes more alkaline due to the proliferation of urease-producing bacteria and/or loss of CO_2
Turbidity	Increase in bacteria and crystals results in a more turbid sample.

Chemical preservation

Chemicals can also be added to preserve the urine sample. Depending on the type of chemical, it may preserve one element but at the expense of another. Common chemical preservatives include acidifiers, formaldehyde, toluene, and commercial chemical urinary preservatives. Note the type of preservation used in the urine sample.

Physical examination of urine

Volume

An accurate representation of urine volume should be assessed over a period of 24 hours. All voided urine is collected and measured to determine if the quantity produced is appropriate. When assessing urine volume, ensure consistency with the patient's regular routine (e.g., regular diet and access to water and regular medications and/or supplements). Factors such as environmental temperature and fluid intake will impact the volume of urine produced. Normal canine and feline urine output ranges from 20 to 40 mL/kg of body weight per day.

Terminology related to urine volume
- Polyuria: increased amounts of urine
- Oliguria: decreased amounts of urine
- Anuria: no urine production
- Pollakiuria: frequent urination
- Dysuria: painful urination

Color

In most species, typical urine color is described as being yellow or straw. The pigment of the urine often correlates with the concentration of the sample, but this should still be confirmed with an SG reading. A low SG is associated with lighter-colored urine, whereas a high SG is associated with darker urine (Table 4.3).

To avoid discrepancies among technicians, use standard color terms when recording your findings.

Table 4.3   Urine color significance

Color	Significance
Colorless or pale	Dilute urine
Deep yellow	Concentrated urine; bilirubinuria
Red to red-brown	Hematuria; hemoglobinuria
Brown	Myoglobinuria
Milky white	Pyuria

Table 4.4   Urine odor significance

Odor	Significance
Ammonia	Cystitis caused by urease-producing bacteria
Fruity/sweet	Ketones
Putrid	Degradation of protein
Strong	Increased concentration; common in intact male cats and goats
Typical	Expected for that species

Odor

The odor of urine can provide insight into possible conditions that should later be confirmed through chemical and sediment analysis (Table 4.4). Urine odor varies with the species as well as gender.

Turbidity

Turbidity refers to the "cloudiness" of urine. An increase in turbidity in the urine can be caused by cellular elements, crystals, microorganisms, or mucus. When examining the turbidity of a sample, there are a few key points to remember.

- Assess turbidity on a fresh sample, at room temperature.
- Ensure that your sample is well mixed by inverting the container several times prior to examination.
- Examine the turbidity in a clear container of a standard depth. A good choice is a urine tube or sterile red-top blood collection tube.
- Horses and rabbits typically have turbid urine caused by mucus and calcium carbonate crystals normally found with those species.

Examining turbidity
(1) With the sample in a standardized, clear tube, invert several times to ensure that the sample is well mixed.
(2) Hold the sample up in front of a piece of paper with text on it.
(3) Assess how clearly the lettering can be viewed through the sample (Figure 4.2).
(4) Record as clear (0), slightly cloudy (1), cloudy (2), or turbid (3).

Specific gravity

Urine specific gravity (USG or SG) is determined by assessing the density of a liquid (in this case, urine) compared with the density of distilled water (Tables 4.5 and 4.6). Specific gravity can be measured using a refractometer (Figure 4.3), a urinometer, reagent strips, or osmolality. Reagent strips are not considered accurate. The most practical and common method in clinics is the use of a refractometer. Refractometers should be used with room temperature urine, as they are calibrated within a specific temperature range. Refractometers calibrated specifically for veterinary species provide a more accurate reading than those which are not.

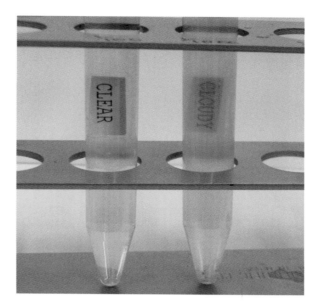

Figure 4.2   Assessing urine turbidity.

Table 4.5   Terms associated with urine specific gravity

Term	SG	Description
Hyposthenuria	<1.008	Renal tubules are actively diluting the urine.
Isosthenuria	1.008–1.012	The urine has not been concentrated or diluted.
Hypersthenuria	>1.012	Renal tubules are concentrating the urine.
Adequate	*See species variations chart*	Urine is being concentrated to an acceptable level to prevent azotemia.

Table 4.6   Urine specific gravity species variation

Species	USG range	Adequate level	Hyposthenuria	Isosthenuria
Canine	1.001–1.065	>1.030	<1.008	1.008–1.012
Feline	1.001–1.080	>1.040	<1.008	1.008–1.012
Bovine	1.005–1.040	>1.025	<1.007	1.008–1.013
Horses	1.020–1.050	>1.025	<1.007	1.008–1.013
Ovine	1.020–1.040	>1.025	<1.007	1.008–1.013

Calibrating the refractometer

Refractometers should be calibrated weekly or daily (depending on use). Apply a drop of room temperature distilled water onto the refractometer. A properly calibrated refractometer should read 1.000 (Figure 4.4). If not, the reading can be adjusted by turning the adjustment screw as directed by the manufacturer.

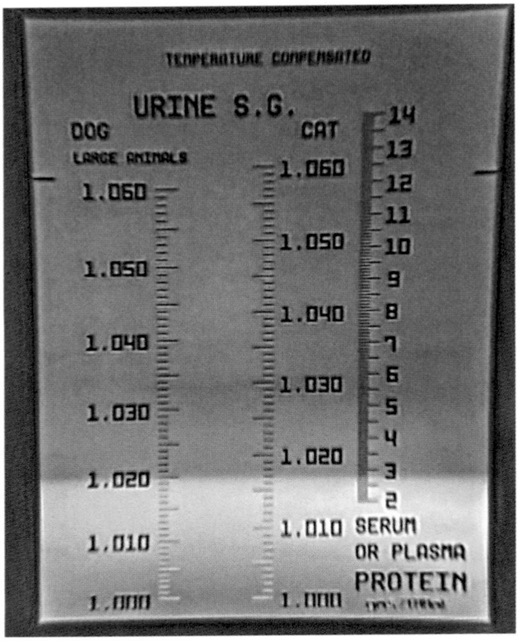

Figure 4.3 Urine specific gravity reading on a refractometer. The reading should be taken where the dark and light areas meet, on the scale appropriate for the species.

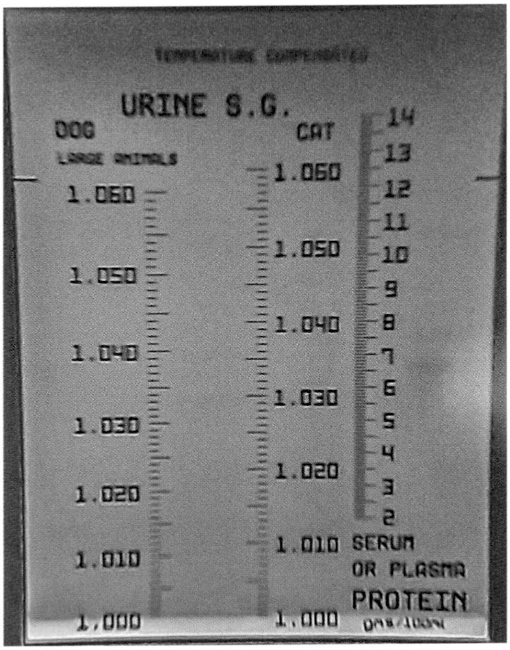

Figure 4.4 Refractometer calibration. The reading for distilled water should be 1.000.

Diluting the sample to accommodate off-scale readings

Depending on the type of refractometer available, as well as the sample being tested, readings may fall above the upper limit of the refractometer.

(1) Dilute the urine 1:1 with distilled water. Mix this dilution in a separate tube or container, not on the surface of the refractometer and not in the main urine container.
(2) Read the SG (e.g., 1.032).
(3) Multiply the last two digits of your reading by 2 (32 × 2 = 64).
(4) Reported the SG reading (1.064).

Chemical examination of urine (stick and tablets)

Determination of chemical constituents of urine can be performed with commercial reagent strips or reagent tablets. The strips are most common and are available with a variety of test pads for different measurements (Figure 4.5). Most chemical reagent strips were developed for human urinalysis testing; therefore, the accuracy and usefulness in veterinary medicine can vary between individual tests. The interpretation and errors pertaining to commercial reagent strips are discussed below.

When using the reagent strips, ensure that each pad is fully saturated with urine and that any excess urine is tapped off, so it does not pool on the pads. This can be

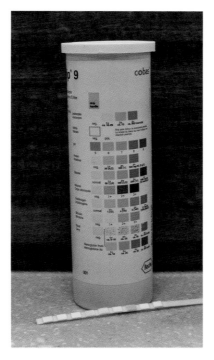

Figure 4.5　Commercial urine chemistry testing strips.

achieved by adding urine to the test strip or by submerging the strip in the urine. Follow the manufacturer's recommendations as to which method is advised. The color change reaction will begin, and results should be compared to a reference color chart, typically found on the side of the strip container or box. Follow the manufacturer's recommendations as to when each reagent pad should be read for color change (Table 4.7).

Table 4.7   Urine chemistry strip interpretation

Constituent	Interpretation	Errors
Glucose (glucosuria, glycosuria) Glucose is a high-level threshold substance and readily reabsorbed in the tubules. Glucosuria occurs when the blood levels of glucose exceed the renal threshold.	Pathologic glucosuria • Diabetes mellitus • Hyperadrenocorticism • Hyperthyroidism Physiologic glucosuria • Fear or stress can result in glucosuria (especially in cats)	False positives • Exposure to oxidizing agents (e.g., hydrogen peroxide and chlorine bleach) False negatives • Formalin • Failure to warm to room temperature
Ketones (ketonuria) Includes acetone, acetoacetic acid and beta-hydroxybutyric acid Ketones are a by-product of fat metabolism. When lipids are used as an energy source (rather than carbohydrates), ketones are produced.	• Uncontrolled diabetes mellitus • Pregnancy toxemia in ruminants • Starvation • Low-carbohydrate diet (high fat and protein)	False positives • Pigmented urine (red) • Highly concentrated urine • Acidic pH False negatives • Aged urine sample (highly volatile) • Bacteriuria
Blood (hematuria, hemoglobinuria, myoglobinuria) *Hematuria* Intact RBCs in the urine *Hemoglobinuria* Free hemoglobin present in the urine *Myoglobinuria* Muscle protein, released from damaged muscle tissue, found in the urine	Hematuria • Indicates bleeding in the urinary tract Hemoglobinuria • Associated with intravascular hemolysis • Dilute or highly alkaline urine can cause red cell lysis in the urine sample Myoglobinuria • Severe skeletal muscle damage. To differentiate hematuria, hemoglobinuria and myoglobinuria see Table 4.10	False positives • Exposure to oxidizing agents (e.g., hydrogen peroxide and chlorine bleach) • Blood contamination of sample False negatives • Poorly mixed urine • Increased SG • Formalin

Table 4.7 *(Continued)*

Constituent	Interpretation	Errors
pH Neutral = 7 Alkaline >7 Acidic <7	Dietary • Herbivores commonly have a pH of >7 (alkaline) • Carnivores and nursing herbivores commonly have a pH of <7 (acidic) Alkaline urine • Urinary tract infections caused by urease-producing bacteria • Urine retention • Drug induced • Alkalosis Acidic urine • Starvation • Fever • Drug induced • Acidosis	• The pH of standing urine will become more alkaline due to the loss of CO_2 as well as the activity of urease-producing bacteria • pH will be falsely low in highly acidic urine due to transfer from the neighboring protein chemical pad
Protein (proteinuria) Normally absent or present in low levels. Protein pad primarily detects albumin.	Transient proteinuria • Stress • Muscle exertion • During estrus • Following parturition Pathologic proteinuria • Acute nephritis • Chronic renal disease • Renal trauma Postrenal proteinuria • Cystitis • Inflammation of genital tract	False positives • Highly alkaline urine • Urine retention False negatives • Low sensitivity to microalbuminuria • Proteinuria caused by nonalbumin sources (globulins or Bence-Jones protein)
Bilirubin (bilirubinuria) Only conjugated bilirubin is found in the urine.	Dogs have a low threshold for bilirubin which can be seen in highly concentrated samples Pathologic causes • Biliary obstruction • Hepatic disease	False positives • Highly pigmented urine • Hemoglobinemia False negatives • Aged urine samples left at room temperature • Exposure to UV light • Ascorbic acid

(Continued)

Table 4.7 (*Continued*)

Constituent	Interpretation	Errors
Urobilinogen Unreliable in veterinary samples	Positive result is insignificant	False positives • Highly pigmented urine • Sulfonamides False negatives • Exposure to UV light • Formalin
Nitrite Unreliable in veterinary samples	• Indirect method of indicating bacteriuria • Always confirm bacteria microscopically	False positives • Darkly pigmented urine • Highly concentrated samples • High levels of ascorbic acid False negatives • Short urine retention times • Bacteria which are present cannot convert nitrate to nitrite
Leukocytes (pyuria) Detects leukocyte esterase activity in granulocytes Unreliable in veterinary samples	• Presumes the presence of WBCs in the urine associated with inflammation or infection in the urinary tract.	False positives • Feline samples • Aged samples • Fecal contamination • Formaldehyde False negatives • Canine samples • Glucosuria

Urine sediment examination

Sediment examination is the third step of a complete urinalysis (Procedure 4.1). A sediment exam not only allows the technician to visualize structures such as cells, crystals, and casts but also serves to confirm suspected findings during the physical and chemical examinations previously conducted (Figure 4.6).

The SG of the sample itself can influence the appearance of some structures, specifically leukocytes and erythrocytes, because of osmosis. In samples with an SG of >1.020, these cells will begin to appear smaller, distorted, and shriveled. In more dilute urine (<1.010), the cells will swell and may eventually rupture given enough time.

Procedure 4.1 Microscopic examination of urine

Materials
- Conical urine tubes
- Centrifuge
- Microscope
- Slides and cover slip
- Sediment stain (if preferred)

Procedure
(1) Pour 5 mL urine into a labeled conical centrifuge tube.
(2) Centrifuge the sample for 5 minutes at 1500 rpm.
(3) Remove the majority of the supernatant while leaving a small amount (0.5–1.0 mL) to resuspend the sediment.
(4) Resuspend the sediment by flicking the tube with your fingers (preferred) or gently mixing the sediment and supernatant with a pipette. The use of a pipette could lead to damage of cellular components.
(5) Using a pipette, transfer a small drop onto a microscope slide and place a coverslip over it (Figure 4.6).
   Optional: If using a sediment stain, transfer a small amount of resuspended sediment to a separate tube as it is good practice to maintain unstained urine. Add 1 or 2 drops of stain. Add a drop of stained urine to the opposite end of the same microscope slide and apply a coverslip.
(6) Decrease the light intensity of the microscope and increase the contrast by lowering the condenser.
(7) Examine a minimum of 10 fields under low power (10×) as well as high power (40×). 10× is used to evaluate larger elements such as casts and large crystals, whereas 40× is used to examine cellular components, infectious agents, and smaller crystals.

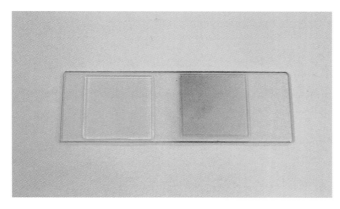

Figure 4.6 Urine sediment prepared for microscopic examination. Unstained (left) and stained (right).

The use of sediment stain is a matter of personal preference (Table 4.8). If it is used, do not mix the stain and sample on the slide. The stain should be mixed with the urine in a separate conical tube and then a drop applied to a slide for examination. Do not stain the entire urine sediment, as some unstained material should be reserved for evaluation.

Reporting of findings

Methods of reporting findings will vary from practice to practice; however, they should be consistent within the practice (Table 4.9)

- Casts are examined and evaluated as the average number seen per low-power (10×) field.
- Red blood cells and white blood cells are evaluated as the average number seen per high-power field (HPF) (40×).
- Other elements, such as bacteria and crystals, are also examined under high power (40×).

Table 4.8   Urine sediment stain considerations

Advantages	Disadvantages
• Provides contrast to microscopic elements, making some easier to visualize	• Introduces artifact and precipitates • Becomes contaminated with bacteria • Dilutes the sample

Best practices when using stain
- Avoid contamination of the bottle tip
- Inspect stain regularly for contamination and precipitates by examining microscopically for the presence of bacteria
- Replace stain regularly
- Prepare a nonstained sample when examining the urine to be used as a comparison to rule out contaminants and artifact

Table 4.9   Examples of enumerating and reporting microscopic findings for WBCS, RBCS, and epithelial cells

No. of cells/HPF		Report as:
None	None observed	None observed
<5	Rare	1+
5–20	Mild	2+
20–100	Moderate	3+
>100	Marked	4+

Urine dry slide examination

Another useful procedure for examining urine sediment is to prepare a dry slide similar to a blood smear (Procedure 4.2). This allows better visualization and differential staining of cellular components in the urine sample. Due to the low protein content of the urine, the sample is prone to washing off the slide during the staining process. To minimize this, ensure that the smear is fully dry (a hair dryer on the low setting can assist with this). Using serum-coated slides can also increase the sample adherence during the staining process.

Procedure 4.2   Urine dry slide preparation

(1) Following centrifugation, place one drop of sediment (unstained) onto a slide and make a smear, similar to how you would do a blood smear.
(2) Allow the smear to fully dry (use a hair dryer on a low setting to assist if needed).
(3) Stain with a quick stain (e.g., Romanowski type, like Diff-Quik).
(4) Allow to air dry and examine under 1000× magnification (Figure 4.7).

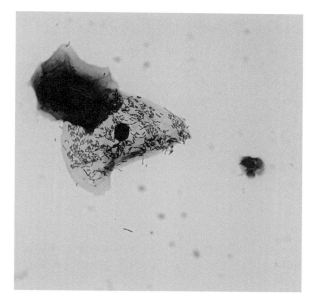

Figure 4.7   Microscopic view of a urine dry slide preparation. Two squamous epithelial cells with adhered bacteria are seen, along with a neutrophil (right).

Microscopic components of urine

Erythrocytes (RBCs)

The presence of fewer than 5 RBCs per HPF is considered acceptable (Figure 4.8). Sample handling and characteristics such as SG and age of the sample can affect the appearance of the RBCs. The presence of erythrocytes can reflect

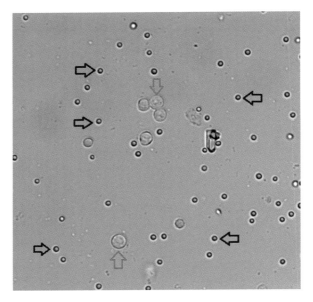

Figure 4.8 Erythrocytes (red arrows) and leukocytes (blue arrows) present in a urine sample (unstained).

contamination of a free-catch sample or may be iatrogenic in the case of cystocentesis and bladder expression. Erythrocytes can also be confused with fat droplets or yeasts. To differentiate them, fat droplets will float in and out of the planes of focus, while RBCs will not. Fat droplets also vary in size. Adding 2% acetic acid to the sample will lyse the RBCs, making evaluation of other components easier. If yeast is suspected, examine closely for the characteristic oval or budding formations.

Microscopic evaluation for the presence of erythrocytes can assist in differentiating between hematuria, hemoglobinuria, and myoglobin (Table 4.10).

Leukocytes (WBCs)

The presence of fewer than 5 WBCs per HPF is considered acceptable (Figure 4.8). The most common leukocyte seen in urine is the neutrophil; however, the findings

Table 4.10 Differentiating hematuria and hemoglobinuria

Condition	Urine color	Supernatant color	Chemical strip reading	Microscopic findings	Plasma
Hematuria	Pink, red, brown	Clear	+	Intact RBCs	Normal
Hemoglobinuria	Pink, red, brown	Unchanged	+	None to few RBCs	Hemolysis
Myoglobin	Red, brown	Unchanged	+	None to few RBCs	Normal

are simply reported as *leukocytes* or *WBCs*. Leukocytes may be confused with renal tubular epithelial cells, which can be differentiated by observing a round nucleus versus the typical segmented nucleus of a neutrophil. The presence of bacteria should also be evaluated when observing leukocytes.

Epithelial cells

Three types of epithelial cells are found in the urinary tract: Squamous epithelial cells, transitional epithelial cells and renal tubular epithelial cells (Table 4.11).

Crystals

Many different types of crystals can be found in the urinary sediment (Table 4.12). Some have clinical significance, while others do not. The presence of crystals in the urine is referred to as crystalluria. Crystals are formed through the precipitation of

Table 4.11   Epithelial cells seen in urine samples

Renal tubular epithelial cells	Transitional epithelial cells	Squamous epithelial cells
Originate from the renal tubules in the kidneys • Round with large, eccentrically located nucleus • Smallest of the epithelial cells • Can be confused with WBCs	Derived from the bladder, ureters, renal pelvis and proximal urethra (mid-urinary tract) • Round, pear shaped, or caudate • often appear like a "fried egg" • Smaller than squamous epithelial cells, but larger than renal tubular cells	Derived from the urethra, prepuce, vagina, and vulva (distal urinary tract) • Partially or fully cornified • Flat, irregularly shaped • Angular borders • May be rolled on themselves
 Figure 4.9 Renal tubular epithelial cell.	 Figure 4.10 Transitional epithelial cell (black arrow). Also present are erythrocytes (red arrows) and a leukocyte (green arrow). Unstained.	 Figure 4.11 Squamous epithelial cells (stained).

Table 4.12   Urinary crystals

Struvite *(magnesium ammonium phosphate; triple phosphate)*	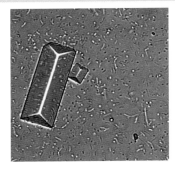 Figure 4.12 Magnesium ammonium phosphate (struvite) crystals.	• Appear as classic "coffin lids"—three- to six-sided colorless prisms usually found in alkaline urine • May be associated with urease-producing bacteria of lower urinary tract disease • Can be associated with triple phosphate uroliths • Readily observed at low magnification
Amorphous phosphate/urates	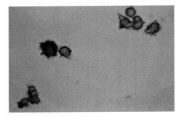 Figure 4.13 Amorphous crystals.	• Phosphates found in alkaline urine appear as a colorless granular precipitate • Urates are similar but are found in acidic urine and are brown • Requires higher magnification
Ammonium urate	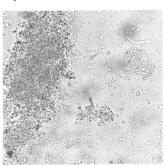 Figure 4.14 Ammonium urate crystals (from McCurnin DM, Bassert JM, *Clinical Textbook for Veterinary Technicians*, 6th ed. St. Louis, MO: Saunders-Elsevier, 2006). *Source:* From McCurnin, Dennis M. and Bassert, Joanna M, (2006), ELSEVIER.	• Ammonium urate crystals are round and brownish, with long spicules, sometimes having a "thorn-apple" or "mange mite" appearance • Seen in liver disease or portocaval shunts • Typically identified at low magnification
Calcium carbonate	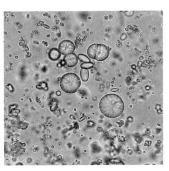 Figure 4.15 Calcium carbonate.	• Often found in horse and rabbit urine • Resemble colorless to yellow-brown dumbbells, oval, wheel-like in shape with radial striations • Easily observed at low magnification

Table 4.12   (*Continued*)

Calcium oxalate dihydrate

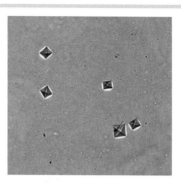

Figure 4.16   Calcium oxalate dihydrate.

- Small, colorless square envelopes, sometimes dumbbell or ring formed, usually with a characteristic "X" in the center
- Can be extremely small, requiring higher magnification
- Generally, in acidic urine, but can be seen in neutral or alkaline urine
- Dihydrate calcium oxalate crystals are found in healthy animals
- Also associated with calcium oxalate urolithiasis
- Occasionally seen in ethylene glycol toxicity

Calcium oxalate monohydrate

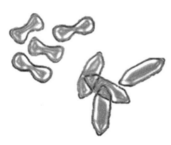

Figure 4.17   Calcium oxalate monohydrate.

- Monohydrate calcium oxalate crystals can be seen in animals with ethylene glycol toxicity, or in large animals that ingested oxalates
- Can be extremely small requiring higher magnification
- Can be seen in urine from healthy horses
- Colorless, often spindle, picket fence slat or hempseed (orzo pasta) shaped. The picket fence and hempseed shapes are more frequently associated with ethylene glycol intoxication

Leucine/cystine/ tyrosine

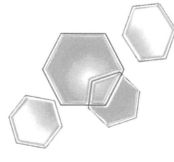

Figure 4.18   Cystine.

- May indicate hepatic disease
- Leucine crystals are small and round, with sectioned centers rarely found in veterinary samples
- Tyrosine crystals appear spiculated and spindle shaped
- Cystine crystals are flat and hexagon shaped
- All three are found in acidic urine
- Cystine crystals almost exclusively found in male dog urine

(*Continued*)

Table 4.12   (*Continued*)

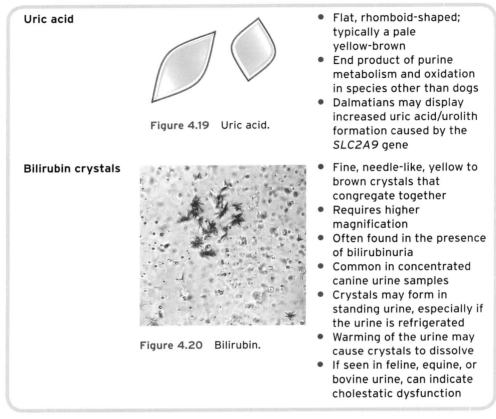

Uric acid

Figure 4.19   Uric acid.

- Flat, rhomboid-shaped; typically a pale yellow-brown
- End product of purine metabolism and oxidation in species other than dogs
- Dalmatians may display increased uric acid/urolith formation caused by the *SLC2A9* gene

Bilirubin crystals

Figure 4.20   Bilirubin.

- Fine, needle-like, yellow to brown crystals that congregate together
- Requires higher magnification
- Often found in the presence of bilirubinuria
- Common in concentrated canine urine samples
- Crystals may form in standing urine, especially if the urine is refrigerated
- Warming of the urine may cause crystals to dissolve
- If seen in feline, equine, or bovine urine, can indicate cholestatic dysfunction

solutes in the urine. A concentrated urine sample or prolonged urine retention increases the likelihood of crystal formation.

Infectious agents

Bacteria
Bacteria seen in a urine sample can indicate bacterial cystitis; however, the collection methods should be taken into consideration. Bacterial contamination is common in voided samples and should be interpreted as such. When bacteria are noted, the shape and arrangement should be documented (Figure 4.24). Further testing, such as Gram staining or a culture and sensitivity, can also be performed.

Fungal organisms
Fungal and yeast organisms may also be seen microscopically. Infections are rare; however, the presence of these organisms should be noted. Contamination by environmental fungal organisms is also a possibility (Figure 4.27).

Parasites
There are parasites which infect the urinary tract, and their ova may be seen during a microscopic examination (Figures 4.25 and 4.26). See Chapter 5 for further descriptions.

Casts

The term cylindruria is used when casts are identified in urine sediment. Casts are formed within the renal tubules and, as a result, reflect the shape of the tubule itself. Casts consist of Tamm-Horsfall protein, which is secreted in the tubules. Other elements may become embedded within the cast, altering its appearance (Table 4.13).

Table 4.13   Urinary casts

Hyaline cast	• Most commonly encountered type of cast • Composed of Tamm-Horsfall mucoprotein • Colorless • More likely to be seen with high proteinuria	 Figure 4.21 Hyaline cast (from Hendrix CM, Sirois M, *Laboratory Procedures for Veterinary Technicians*, 5th ed. St. Louis, MO: Mosby-Elsevier, 2007).
Epithelial cast	• Composed of renal tubular epithelial cells found within the nephron • RTE cells slough off of the walls of the tubules and become embedded in the cast • Can result from acute tubular injury such as severe dehydration	 Figure 4.22 Epithelial cast (from Hendrix CM, Sirois M, *Laboratory Procedures for Veterinary Technicians*, 5th ed. St. Louis, MO: Mosby-Elsevier, 2007).
RBC cast	• RBCs are embedded in the cast when hemorrhage occurs in the tubule • Red-orange	
WBC cast	• WBCs produced as a result of inflammation in the tubules will become embedded in the cast (i.e., pyelonephritis) • Neutrophils are the typical WBCs in the cast but can be mistaken for granular casts due to degradation of the WBCs • Staining will enhance nuclear detail	

(Continued)

Table 4.13 (*Continued*)

Granular cast	<ul><li>Both coarse and fine granular casts can be seen</li><li>Is a result of degradation of cellular elements in the cast matrix</li><li>Can be mistaken for amorphous debris/clumps</li></ul>	

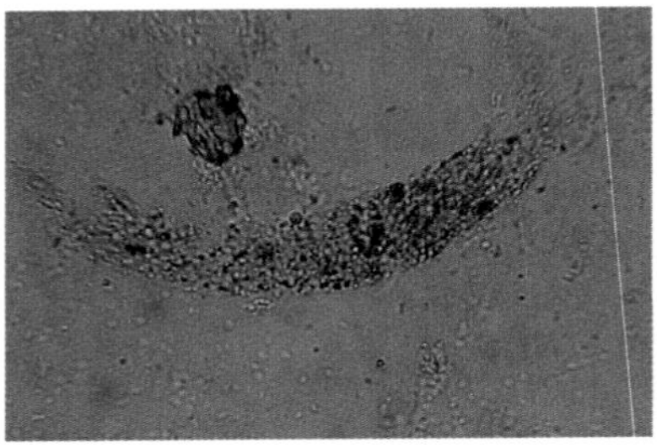

Figure 4.23 Granular cast (from Hendrix CM, Sirois M, *Laboratory Procedures for Veterinary Technicians*, 5th ed. St. Louis, MO: Mosby-Elsevier, 2007). *Source:* From Hendrix, Charles M. and Sirois, Margi, (2007), ELSEVIER.

Waxy cast	<ul><li>A natural progression following the further degradation of granular casts</li><li>Casts have a waxy appearance and can be yellow or colorless, with jagged, irregular edges</li><li>Can indicate more chronic tubular injury</li></ul>
Fatty cast	<ul><li>Contains fat droplets within the protein matrix</li><li>Fat droplets are highly refractile</li><li>May be normal in small numbers in cats</li></ul>

Artifacts

Depending on the method of collection, various artifacts can be seen within the sediment and should be disregarded, as they are not considered pathogenic (Table 4.14). Pollen, hair, and environmental yeast are common artifacts seen in urine collected while the animal is walking outside. Starch crystals (talcum) from gloves can contaminate a sample, giving the appearance of crystalluria (Figure 4.31).

Table 4.14 Infectious agents and artifacts

Infectious agents	Artifacts and other findings

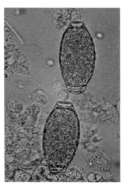

Figure 4.29 Spermatozoa (black arrows). Also present are erythrocytes (blue arrows) and a leukocyte (red arrow).

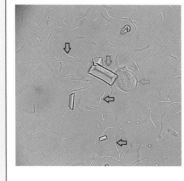

Figure 4.28 Mucus strand (black arrow). Also present are squamous epithelial cells (blue arrows).

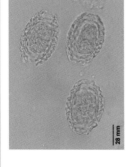

Figure 4.25 *Dioctophyma renale* ovum (from Zajac AM, Conboy GA, *Veterinary Clinical Parasitology*, 8th ed. Ames, IA: Blackwell Publishing, 2012). *Source:* From Zajac, Anne M. and Conboy, Gary A, (2012), John Wiley & Sons.

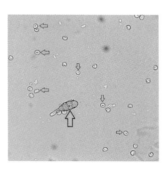

Figure 4.31 Artifact (starch granules).

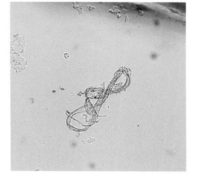

Figure 4.30 Artifact (fibers).

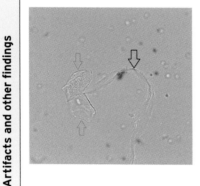

Figure 4.27 Fungal organisms (black arrow). Also present are multiple erythrocytes (red arrows).

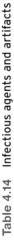

Figure 4.24 Bacilli bacteria (black arrows). Also present are struvite crystals (red arrow) and a transitional epithelial cell (blue arrow).

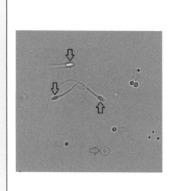

Figure 4.26 *Pearsonema plica* ovum (from Hendrix CM, Robinson E, *Diagnostic Parasitology for Veterinary Technicians*, 4th ed. St. Louis, MO: Mosby-Elsevier, 2012). *Source:* From Hendrix, Charles M. and Robinson, (2012), ELSEVIER.

Chapter 5
Parasitology

Parasites can inhabit any body system and may be benign or detrimental. Experience observing different body fluids, samples, and skin scrapings can greatly enhance the likelihood of correctly identifying parasitic infections (inside the body) and infestations (outside the body). Spurious infections (evidence of a parasite within a non-host animal) can also be encountered, and correct diagnosis of a true infection is necessary to render the appropriate treatment, if any. With the development of parasite resistance to medications, proper identification is critical so a targeted and effective treatment may be administered. Additionally, there is zoonotic potential with many veterinary parasites, which makes accurate identification an important step for human safety.

There are geographic differences as to the prevalence of certain parasites. Not all parasites are represented in this chapter; the focus is on parasites frequently encountered in North America.

Sample collection and handling

Skin samples

Skin scrapings
The skin scraping technique is used to evaluate a sample for external parasites, specifically burrowing mites. To increase the likelihood of obtaining a diagnostic sample, the targeted collection area should be a zone where affected areas and unaffected areas meet. Refer to the "Scrapings" section of the cytology chapter for materials and procedures.

The suspected parasite will determine the depth of scraping needed. For example, burrowing mites such as *Demodex* spp. require a scraping to a depth where a small amount of capillary blood begins to be produced.

Cellophane tape preparation
The cellophane tape preparation method is ideal for collecting surface parasites such as lice and surface (nonburrowing) mites (Procedure 5.1).

Veterinary Technician's Handbook of Laboratory Procedures, Second Edition. Brianne Bellwood and Melissa Andrasik-Catton.
© 2023 John Wiley & Sons, Inc. Published 2023 by John Wiley & Sons, Inc.
Companion website: www.wiley.com/go/bellwoodhandbook2

Procedure 5.1 Cellophane tape preparation

Materials
- Clear cellophane tape
- Mineral oil
- Microscope slide

Procedure
(1) Part the fur if needed to access the skin surface.
(2) Press the cellophane tape onto the skin (sticky side down) and lift (Figure 5.1).
(3) Add a couple of drops of mineral oil to a microscope slide.
(4) Place the tape onto the slide (sticky side down).
(5) Examine using 40× magnification.

Blood samples

When examining for blood parasites, collection into an EDTA blood tube is preferred if collecting a blood sample directly onto the slide is not possible. If serum or plasma is required for immunologic tests, then a red-top (no anticoagulant) or green-top (heparin) tube is required. Review the package insert of serological test kits or the reference laboratory guidelines to ensure proper sample type and volume.

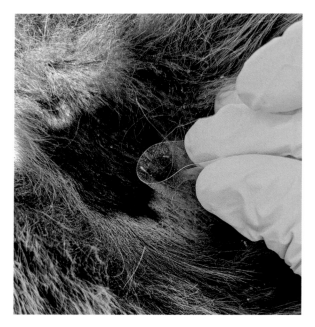

Figure 5.1 Using clear cellophane tape to collect samples for examination of surface parasites.

Urine, respiratory, and other system samples

The collection of samples from other body systems is very specific and encompasses a range of materials and methods for sampling, handling, and storage. Urine sediment can be microscopically reviewed for presence of parasitic ova and reported during a routine urinalysis. Refer to the urinalysis chapter for materials and methods. Methods of obtaining samples from other areas, such as the respiratory tract, are outside the scope of this book and should be discussed with the veterinarian.

Fecal samples

Fecal samples collected should be fresh; however, if that is not possible, preservation methods should be used. Refrigeration or the use of 10% formalin (1:1 ratio) can prevent or delay the development of the ova. Freezing can be done, but the ova of certain parasites (e.g., strongyle type) may not be recoverable in representative quantities.

For small animal fecal samples, a minimum of 1 g, preferably 2 g, of fresh feces should be collected. For best results, samples from different areas of the feces should be collected. Small samples obtained directly from the animal using a gloved finger or a fecal loop can be examined; however, they are often suitable only for a direct smear, as the amount collected is quite small.

For large animal fecal samples, feces may be obtained directly from the rectum of an individual animal or multiple animals from the same pen or pasture to obtain a pooled sample. Pooled samples provide insight to the overall parasite load of a group of animals housed together. When collecting a pooled sample, pay close attention to individuals that are displaying symptoms of high parasite load (e.g., poor body condition).

Diagnostic procedures of parasites of the gastrointestinal tract

Gross examination

Prior to isolation of parasite ova, the feces should be examined to note the following characteristics.
(1) Consistency
(2) Color
(3) Presence of blood or mucus
(4) Presence of foreign bodies
(5) Presence of adult parasites or tapeworm proglottids

Microscopic examination

Direct smear
The direct smear evaluation can be made on fecal, sputum, urine, and blood specimens to scan for parasite larvae and parasite ova. This method requires little equipment; however, due to the small sample size, a direct smear alone is not adequate to detect parasites which are present in lower numbers (Procedure 5.2).

Figure 5.2   Direct fecal smear.

Procedure 5.2   Direct fecal smear

Materials
- Wooden applicator stick
- Saline
- Microscope slides
- Cover slips

Procedure
(1) Using the wooden applicator stick, collect a small amount of feces. Only a small amount should coat the stick.
(2) Add 1 drop of saline to a microscope slide.
    If body fluids are being tested, mix directly with the saline on the slide.
(3) Mix the feces into the saline with the applicator stick. The goal is to make a thin emulsion, free of any clumps or large pieces of material (Figure 5.2).
(4) Apply a coverslip.
(5) Examine the entire slide under 100× and 400× magnification for the presence of ova, larvae, cysts and trophozoites.

Ovum concentration techniques

Fecal flotation
Flotation methods rely on the differences in specific gravity of the parasite ova and the fecal debris (Procedure 5.3). A flotation solution should permit the ova to float to the surface while causing other fecal material to sink. There are a number of flotation solutions available, each with its own advantages and disadvantages (Table 5.1).

Procedure 5.3   Simple flotation technique

Materials
- Shell vial
- Flotation solution
- Coverslip
- Microscope slide
- Tongue depressor

Table 5.1   Fecal flotation solutions

Flotation solution	Ingredients	Advantages/disadvantages
Magnesium sulfate	350 g $MgSO_4$ (Epsom salt) 1000 mL water	Corrosive; forms crystals
Sheather's solution (sugar solution)	454 g granulated sugar 355 mL water 6 mL of 40% formaldehyde per 100 mL of solution as a preservative	Messy to work with; does not distort nematode ova; inexpensive
Saturated salt	350 g NaCl (table salt) 1000 mL water	Forms crystals; heavy ovum distortion; corrosive
Sodium nitrate	315 g $NaNO_3$ 1000 mL water	Forms crystals; ovum distortion occurs after 20 minutes
Zinc sulfate	386 g of $ZnSO_4$ 1000 mL water	Some trematode ova will not float

- Sample cup
- Tea strainer (or gauze or cheesecloth)

Procedure
(1) Add approximately 2 g (1/2 tsp) of feces to a sample cup.
(2) Add 20-30 mL of flotation solution.
(3) Using a tongue depressor, mix the solution until it becomes homogeneous.
(4) Filter the solution through a tea strainer.
(5) Add this filtered solution to a shell vial until it forms a meniscus. If there isn't enough filtered solution to fill the shell, add more flotation solution until a positive meniscus is formed.
(6) Place a glass coverslip over the meniscus.
(7) Allow the sample to sit undisturbed for 10-20 minutes (Figure 5.3).

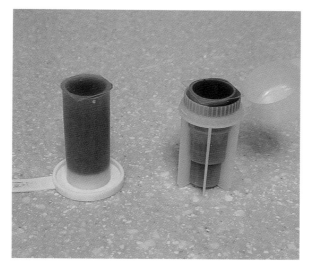

Figure 5.3   Simple float technique. Various styles of "shells" are commercially available.

(8) Carefully remove the coverslip by lifting it directly upwards (do not tip to the side) and place it onto a microscope slide.
Placing the coverslip down at a slight angle will help to push out air bubbles
(9) Examine the entire area using 100×-400× magnification.

Centrifugation technique

The centrifugation technique provides a more efficient method of parasite ovum recovery than the simple flotation method (Procedure 5.4). A variable-angle centrifuge with swinging buckets is preferred for this procedure.

Procedure 5.4   Centrifugation technique

Materials
● Conical, centrifuge tubes
● Flotation solution
● Coverslip
● Microscope slide
● Tongue depressor
● Sample cup
● Tea strainer (or gauze or cheesecloth)

Procedure
(1) Add approximately 2 g (1/2 tsp) of feces to a sample cup.
(2) Add 20-30 mL of flotation solution.
(3) Using a tongue depressor, mix the solution until it becomes homogeneous.
(4) Filter the solution through a tea strainer.
(5) Add this filtered solution to a centrifuge tube.
(6) Top up with flotation solution until a positive meniscus is formed.
(7) Apply a coverslip (Figure 5.4).

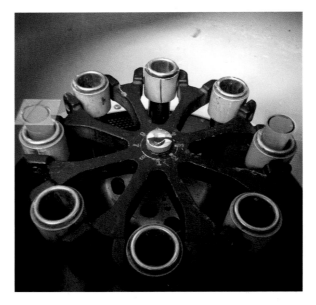

Figure 5.4   Tube placement for centrifugation technique.

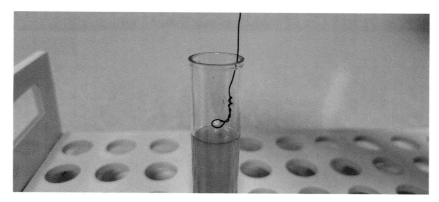

Figure 5.5 Collection of surface material using a wire loop following centrifugation.

(8) Centrifuge for 5 minutes at 1500 rpm.
(9) Carefully remove the coverslip and add to a microscope slide as described in the simple flotation procedure.
(10) Examine the entire area using 100×–400× magnification.

Alternative method
In some cases, the coverslip may not adhere to the tube during the centrifugation process. A modification of the technique described above can be used. This alternative method can also be used if a variable angle centrifuge is not available. Complete steps 1 to 5 as described above.

(1) Centrifuge for 5 minutes at 1500 rpm.
(2) Without disturbing the tubes, use a wire loop (bent at 90°) to gently collect surface material from the centrifuged sample (Figure 5.5).
(3) Transfer this to a microscope slide and add a coverslip.
(4) Examine the entire area using 100×–400× magnification.

Sedimentation technique
The sedimentation technique is used when parasite ova are too large and heavy to be effectively recovered using flotation techniques (e.g., fluke ova). One disadvantage to this technique is the increased amount of fecal debris that will be present during examination.

Procedure 5.5   Fecal sedimentation technique

Materials
- Conical centrifuge tubes
- Distilled water
- Coverslip
- Microscope slide
- Tongue depressor
- Pipettes
- Sample cup
- Tea strainer (or gauze or cheesecloth)

Procedure
(1) Add approximately 2 g (1/2 tsp) of feces to a sample cup.
(2) Add 20–30 mL of distilled water.
(3) Using a tongue depressor, mix the solution until it becomes homogeneous.
(4) Filter the solution through a tea strainer.
(5) Centrifuge the sample for 5 minutes at 1500 rpm. (If a centrifuge is not available, allow the sample to sit for 20–30 minutes.)
(6) Decant the supernatant without disturbing the sediment.
(7) Using a pipette, transfer a small amount of the upper layer of sediment to a microscope slide. Dilute as needed.
(8) Apply a coverslip.
(9) Repeat step 7 with the bottom layer of sediment.
(10) Examine both preparations using 100×–400× magnification.

Quantitative methods

Quantitative methods (e.g., McMaster or Wisconsin technique) are used to determine the number of ova or cysts per gram of feces (Procedure 5.6). It provides a rough estimate of the level of parasite load; however, there are many factors that affect egg detection, and therefore, the results may not fully represent the parasite burden of an individual animal.

Procedure 5.6   McMaster technique

Materials
- McMaster egg counting chamber slides (Figure 5.6)
- Sample cups
- Scale
- Pipettes
- Tea strainer (or gauze or cheesecloth)
- Flotation solution

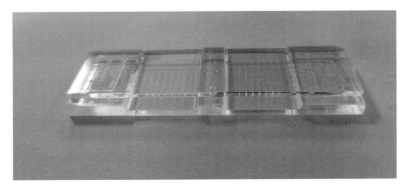

Figure 5.6   McMaster egg counting slide.

Procedure
(1) Using a scale, weigh 2 g of feces.
(2) Mix with 28 mL of flotation solution until it is homogeneous. There are numerous dilution procedures used for sedimentation preparation; follow a consistent procedure within your clinic.
(3) Filter the solution through the tea strainer.
(4) While mixing the filtered solution, obtain a sample using a pipette and transfer it to one of the chambers on the McMaster slide.
(5) Repeat the procedure to fill the other chamber.
(6) Allow the slide to sit for 5 minutes, then count the total number of eggs in both etched grid areas. Keep a separate count for each egg type.
(7) To calculate number of eggs/gram of feces, multiply the total number of eggs counted in the 2 chambers by 50 and report as eggs per gram (e.p.g.). Depending on your feces-to-water dilution ratio, the multiplier may be different.

Other testing methods

Baermann technique
The Baermann technique is a useful method for isolating certain nematode (e.g., roundworm) larvae from feces by encouraging their emergence from their ova (Procedure 5.7). This method is often utilized for isolating lungworm larvae.

Procedure 5.7   Baermann technique

Materials
- Ring stand
- Funnel
- Tea strainer or wire screen
- Rubber tubing
- Clamp
- Cheesecloth or gauze square
- Pipettes
- Conical tube
- Microscope slide
- Coverslip

Procedure
(1) Construct the Baermann apparatus by placing the funnel into the ring apparatus and attach rubber tubing to the end.
(2) Place a tea strainer on top of the funnel and line with a couple of layers of cheesecloth or gauze squares.
(3) Apply clamps at the end of the rubber tubing. Everything should be watertight. Test with water prior to testing samples to ensure a good seal.
(4) Add 15 g of feces to the lined tea strainer.
(5) Cover with warm water (not hot) until the fecal sample is submerged.
(6) Allow the sample to sit overnight to allow the larvae to emerge and sink to the bottom of the tubing.

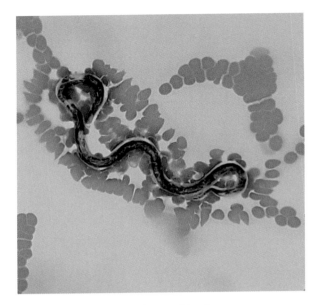

Figure 5.7   Microfilaria of *Dirofilaria immitis* on a blood smear.

(7) Release the clamp slowly and collect a few drops into a conical tube.
(8) Apply one drop to a microscope slide and cover with a coverslip.
(9) Examine the slide for the presence of larvae. Lugol's iodine may be used to stain the larvae for better viewing.
(10) Repeat this several times.

Diagnostic procedures for parasites in other body systems

Whole blood can be used to examine for parasites, such as *Dirofilaria immitis*, by preparing a direct smear or a stained blood smear using EDTA blood (Figure 5.7). The buffy coat layer of a packed cell volume tube will provide a concentration of microfilaria and can increase the likelihood of isolating the parasites (see the hematology chapter for guidelines on preparing a packed cell volume). When looking for intra- or extracellular blood parasites, making a smear directly from freshly collected blood is preferred, as no interference from an anticoagulant has occurred. It is known that *Mycoplasma* species can fall off the RBCs in the presence of EDTA. Refer to the hematology chapter for blood parasite identification.

Modified Knott's technique

The modified Knott's technique (Procedure 5.8) is another method of identifying microfilariae in a blood sample for visual confirmation of the parasite's presence (Table 5.2).

Procedure 5.8   Modified Knott's technique

Materials
- Whole-blood sample
- 2% formalin (2 mL of 40% formaldehyde + 98 mL distilled water)

Table 5.2 Appearance of *Dirofilaria immitis*

Body shape	Straight
Length	310 μm
Head	Tapered

- Conical centrifuge tube
- Methylene blue stain
- Microscope slide
- Coverslip

Procedure

(1) Mix 1 mL of whole blood with 9 mL of 2% formalin. Invert the tube gently several times to lyse the RBCs.
(2) Centrifuge the tube for 5 minutes at 1500 rpm.
(3) Pour off all the supernatant, leaving only sediment.
(4) Add 1 drop of methylene blue stain to the sediment.
(5) Transfer a drop onto a microscope slide and coverslip.
(6) Examine under 100× magnification.

Immunologic tests

Approximately 25% of dogs will have an occult heartworm infection, meaning they do not have circulating microfilaria. This can occur if the infection consists of young heartworms or single-sex parasites. Immunologic tests designed to detect *D. immitis* antigens are preferred as a diagnostic tool. Additionally, they provide an increased level of sensitivity.

Common internal parasites (endoparasites) of domestic species

Nematodes

Adult nematodes, commonly known as roundworms, possess an elongated body which lacks segments and is rounded at each end (Figure 5.8). Their cross-section shape is cylindrical, not flattened as with the cestodes or trematodes. The life cycle of a nematode may or may not involve an intermediate host.

Some nematodes may also produce unique larval stages for identification, such as lungworm larvae (e.g., *Filaroides osleri*) and microfilariae (e.g., *Dirofilaria immitis)*

The nematodes are split into several different superfamilies, which have similar properties and life cycles.

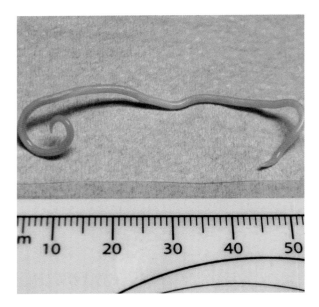

Figure 5.8   Adult nematode (*Toxocara canis*).

Nematodes of dogs and cats

Table 5.3   Ascaridoidea (ascarids) of dogs and cats

Parasite	Definitive host(s)	Common name	Transmission route	Intermediate host	Distribution	Testing method
Toxocara canis (Figure 5.9)	Canine	Roundworm	Egg ingestion	None	Worldwide	Fecal flotation
Toxocara cati (Figure 5.10)	Feline	Roundworm	Egg ingestion	None	Worldwide	Fecal flotation
Toxascaris leonina (Figure 5.11)	Canine and feline	Roundworm	Egg ingestion	None	Worldwide	Fecal flotation

Table 5.4   Dog and cat ascarid comparison

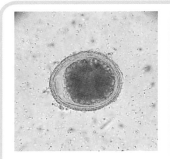
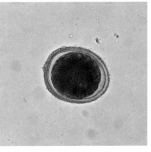
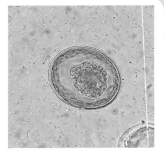

Figure 5.9   *Toxocara canis.*   Figure 5.10   *Toxocara cati.*   Figure 5.11   *Toxascaris leonina.*

Table 5.5 Ancylostomatidae of dogs and cats

Parasite	Definitive host(s)	Common name	Transmission routes	Intermediate host	Distribution	Testing method
Ancylostoma caninum (Figure 5.12)	Canine	Canine hookworm	Egg ingestion; through skin; placental; mammary	None	Worldwide	Fecal flotation
Ancylostoma tubaeforme	Feline	Feline hookworm	Egg ingestion; through skin; placental; mammary	None	Worldwide	Fecal flotation
Ancylostoma braziliense	Canine and feline	Canine and feline hookworm	Egg ingestion; through skin; placental; mammary	None	Worldwide	Fecal flotation
Uncinaria stenocephala	Canine and feline	Northern canine hookworm	Egg ingestion; through skin; placental; mammary	None	North America	Fecal flotation

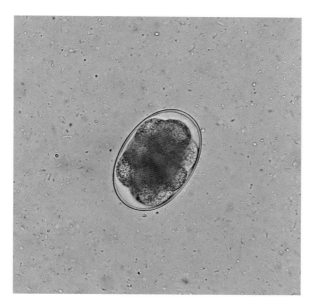

Figure 5.12 *Ancylostoma caninum.*

Table 5.6 Rhabditoidea of dogs and cats

Parasite	Definitive host	Common name	Transmission route	Intermediate host	Distribution	Testing method
Strongyloides stercoralis	Canine	Intestinal threadworm	Through skin; mammary	None	Worldwide	Fecal flotation
Strongyloides tumefaciens	Feline	Intestinal threadworm	Through skin; mammary	None	Worldwide	Fecal flotation

Table 5.7 Metastrongyloidea of dogs and cats

Parasite	Definitive host	Common name	Transmission route	Intermediate host	Distribution	Testing method
Filaroides (Oslerus) osleri	Canine	Canine lungworm	Ingestion of L1 larvae	None	North American, Europe, Japan	Baermann technique
Filaroides hirthi	Canine	Canine lungworm	Same as above	Same as above	Same as above	Same as above
Filaroides milksi	Canine	Canine lungworm	Same as above	Same as above	Same as above	Same as above
Aelurostrongylus abstrusus	Feline	Feline lungworm	Same as above	Same as above	Worldwide	Same as above

Table 5.8 Trichuroidea of dogs and cats

Parasite	Definitive host	Common name	Transmission route	Intermediate host	Distribution	Testing method
Trichuris vulpis (Figure 5.13)	Canine	Canine whipworm	Ingestion of eggs	None	Worldwide	Fecal flotation
Trichuris campanula	Feline	Feline whipworm	Ingestion of eggs	None	Rare in North America	Fecal flotation
Pearsonema plica (Figure 4.26)	Canine	Canine bladder worm	Ingestion of infective intermediate host	Earthworm	Southeastern U.S.	Examination of urine
Pearsonema feliscati	Feline	Feline bladder worm	Ingestion of infective intermediate host	Earthworm	Southeastern U.S.	Examination of urine

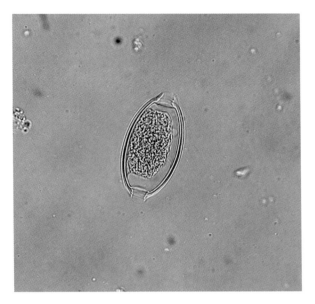

Figure 5.13   *Trichuris* spp.

Table 5.9   Dioctophymoidea of dogs

Parasite	Definitive host	Common name	Transmission route	Intermediate host	Distribution	Testing method
Dioctophyma renale (Figure 5.14)	Canine	Giant kidney worm	Ingestion of infective intermediate host	Annelid worm	North America, Europe	Fecal sedimentation

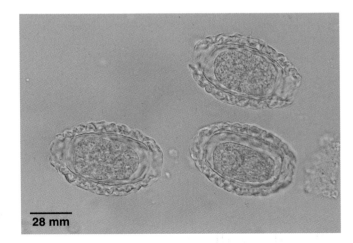
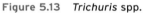

28 mm

Figure 5.14   *Dioctophyma renale* ovum (from Zajac AM, Conboy GA, *Veterinary Clinical Parasitology*, 8th ed. Ames, IA: Blackwell Publishing, 2012). *Source:* From Zajac, Anne M. and Conboy, Gary A, (2012), John Wiley & Sons.

Table 5.10 Filaroidea of dogs and cats

Parasite	Definitive hosts	Common name	Transmission route	Intermediate host	Distribution	Testing method
Dirofilaria immitis (Figure 5.7)	Canine and feline	Heartworm	Bite of infective mosquito	Mosquito	Worldwide (warm climates)	Blood smear; buffy coat examination; modified Knott's technique; immunologic testing

Table 5.11 Ascaridoidea (ascarids) of equines

Parasite	Definitive host	Common name	Transmission route	Intermediate host	Distribution	Testing method
Parascaris equorum (Figure 5.15)	Equine	Equine roundworm	Ingestion of eggs	None	Worldwide	Fecal flotation

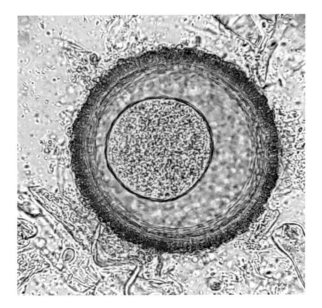

Figure 5.15 *Parascaris equorum.*

Nematodes of equines

Table 5.12 Strongyloidea of equines

Parasite	Definitive host	Common name	Transmission route	Intermediate host	Distribution	Testing method
Strongylus vulgaris (Figure 5.16)	Equine	Strongyles	Ingestion of infective larvae	None	Worldwide	Fecal flotation
Strongylus edentatus	Equine	Strongyles	Ingestion of infective larvae	None	Worldwide	Fecal flotation
Strongylus equinus	Equine	Strongyles	Ingestion of infective larvae	None	Worldwide	Fecal flotation

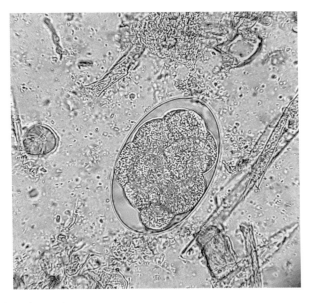

Figure 5.16 Equine strongyle ovum.

Table 5.13 Rhabditoidea of equines

Parasite	Definitive host	Common name	Transmission route	Intermediate host	Distribution	Testing method
Strongyloides westeri (Figure 5.17)	Equine	Intestinal threadworm of horses	Mammary; skin	None	Worldwide	Fecal flotation

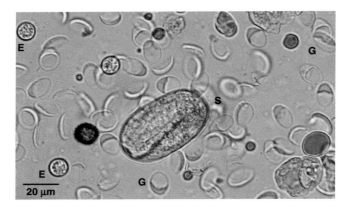

Figure 5.17 Larvated *Strongyloides* egg (S); collapsed *Giardia* cysts (G); *Eimeria* oocysts (E) (from Zajac AM, Conboy GA, *Veterinary Clinical Parasitology*, 8th ed. Ames, IA: Blackwell Publishing, 2012). *Source:* From Zajac, Anne M. and Conboy, Gary A, (2012), John Wiley & Sons.

Table 5.14 Oxyuroidea of equines

Parasite	Definitive host	Common name	Transmission route	Intermediate host	Distribution	Testing method
Oxyuris equi (Figure 5.18)	Equine	Pinworm of horses	Ingestion of eggs	None	Worldwide	Cellophane tape collection of surfaces of the anus; fecal flotation

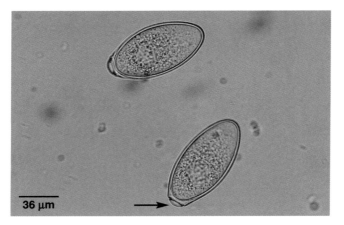

Figure 5.18 *Oxyuris* ova (from Zajac AM, Conboy GA, *Veterinary Clinical Parasitology*, 8th ed. Ames, IA: Blackwell Publishing, 2012). *Source:* From Zajac, Anne M. and Conboy, Gary A, (2012), John Wiley & Sons.

Table 5.15 Spiruroidea of equines

Parasite	Definitive host	Common name	Transmission route	Intermediate host	Distribution	Testing method
Habronema sp. and *Draschia megastoma* larval stages	Equine	Summer sores	Infective larvae deposited into skin wounds by intermediate host (aberrant larvae)	Muscid flies (house fly; face fly)	Worldwide	Skin biopsy
Habronema sp. and *Draschia megastoma* adult parasites	Equine	Stomach worms of horses	Ingestion of infected intermediate host	Muscid flies (house fly; face fly)	Worldwide	Fecal flotation
Thelazia lacrymalis	Equine	Eyeworm of horses	Infective larvae deposited by intermediate host	*Musca autumnalis* (face fly)	Worldwide	Microscopic exam of lacrimal secretions

Nematodes of ruminants

Table 5.16 Trichostrongyloidea of ruminants

Parasite	Definitive host	Common name	Transmission route	Intermediate host	Distribution	Testing method
Bunostomum spp., *Cooperia* spp., *Chabertia* spp., *Haemonchus* spp., *Oesophagostomum* spp., *Trichostrongylus* spp. (Figure 5.19)	Ruminant	Trichostrongyles	Egg ingestion	None	Worldwide	Fecal flotation (trichostrongyle-type egg); unable to differentiate between species microscopically
Nematodirus spp. and *Marshallagia* spp. (Figure 5.20)	Ruminant	Trichostrongyles with large eggs	Egg ingestion	None	Worldwide	Fecal flotation
Dictyocaulus spp.	Ruminant	Lungworms of ruminants	Ingestion of infective larvae	None	Worldwide	Microscopic exam of sputum

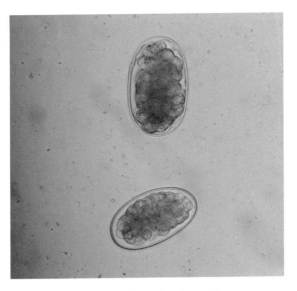

Figure 5.19   *Trichostrongylus* spp. from a sheep fecal sample.

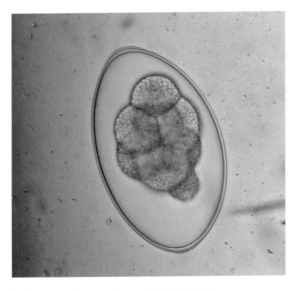

Figure 5.20   *Nematodirus* spp. from a sheep fecal sample.

Table 5.17   Metastrongyloidea of ruminants

Parasite	Definitive hosts	Common name	Transmission route	Intermediate host	Distribution	Testing method
Muellerius capillaris	Sheep and goats	Hair lungworm	Ingestion of infective larvae	None	Worldwide	Larvae identification in fecal flotation

Table 5.18   Trichuroidea of ruminants

Parasite	Definitive hosts	Common name	Transmission route	Intermediate host	Distribution	Testing method
Trichuris ovis (Figure 5.21)	Ruminants	Ruminant whipworm	Egg ingestion	None	Worldwide	Fecal flotation

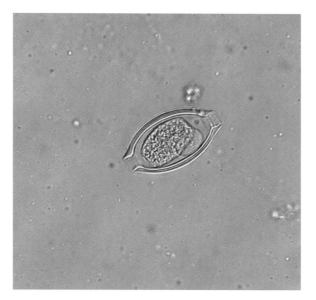

Figure 5.21   *Trichuris ovis.*

Cestodes

Cestodes (tapeworms) differ from nematodes in that they are flattened and segmented. These segments, called proglottids, become more developed towards the distal end of the parasite. These gravid proglottids will contain the tapeworm eggs.

Cestodes require an intermediate host in which development into a larval stage, called a metacestode, occurs. The metacestode often takes the form of a cyst, present in various tissues of the intermediate host. The host becomes infected by ingesting the metacestode larvae in the intermediate host. In some cases, the metacestode stage within the intermediate host is more pathogenic than the mature cestode in the definitive host (e.g., *Taenia solium*) (see Table 5.22).

Table 5.19   Cestodes of dogs and cats

Parasite	Definitive host(s)	Common name	Intermediate hosts	Distribution	Testing method
Dipylidium caninum (Figure 5.22)	Canine and feline	Double-pored tapeworm	Adult fleas (Figure 5.23)	Worldwide	Fecal flotation or opening of dried gravid proglottids to release the egg packet to examine microscopically
Taenia pisiformis	Canine	Canine tapeworm	Rabbits	Worldwide	Fecal flotation or opening of dried gravid proglottids to release embryos
Taenia hydatigena	Canine	Canine tapeworm	Ruminants	Worldwide	Same as above
Taenia ovis	Canine	Mutton tapeworm of dogs	Sheep	Worldwide	Same as above
Taenia taeniaeformis	Feline	Feline tapeworm	Rats and mice	Worldwide	Same as above
Taenia (Multiceps) multiceps (Figure 5.24)	Canine	Coenurus tapeworm	Sheep	Worldwide	Fecal flotation
Taenia serialis	Canine	Canine tapeworm	Rabbits	Worldwide	Fecal flotation
Echinococcus granulosus (Table 5.23)	Canine	Unilocular hydatid tapeworm	Sheep, cattle, and humans	Worldwide	Fecal flotation
Echinococcus multilocularis (Table 5.23)	Feline	Multilocular hydatid tapeworm	Rats, mice, voles, and humans	Northern hemisphere	Fecal flotation

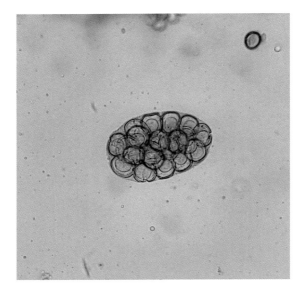

Figure 5.22   *Dipylidium caninum* ova.

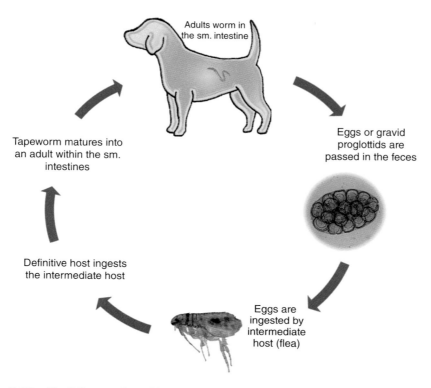

Figure 5.23 *Dipylidium caninum* life cycle.

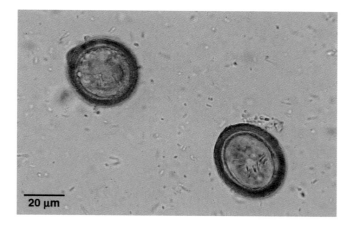

Figure 5.24 *Taenia* sp. ova (from Zajac AM, Conboy GA, *Veterinary Clinical Parasitology*, 8th ed. Ames, IA: Blackwell Publishing, 2012). *Source:* From Zajac, Anne M. and Conboy, Gary A, (2012), John Wiley & Sons.

Table 5.20   Cestodes of equines

Parasite	Definitive host	Common name	Intermediate host	Distribution	Testing method
Anoplocephala spp. and *Paranoplocephala mamillana*	Equine	Equine tapeworm	Grain mite	Worldwide	Fecal flotation

Table 5.21   Cestodes of ruminants

Parasite	Definitive host(s)	Common name	Intermediate host	Distribution	Testing method
Moniezia benedeni	Cattle	Ruminant tapeworm	Grain mite	Worldwide	Fecal flotation
Moniezia expansa (Figure 5.25)	Cattle, sheep, and goats	Ruminant tapeworm	Grain mite	Worldwide	Fecal flotation

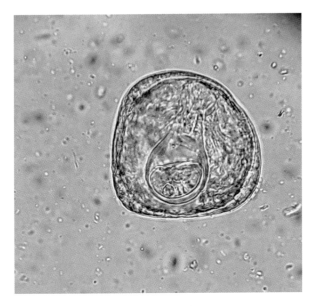

Figure 5.25   *Moniezia* spp. from a sheep fecal sample.

Table 5.22 Metacestode (cystic) stage concerns

Metacestode stage	Intermediate host	Adult cestode	Definitive host(s)	Concerns
Cysticercus cellulosae	Pigs	*Taenia solium*	Humans	"Pork measles" • Humans become infected by ingesting the *C. cellulosae* in undercooked meat. • Cysticercus can develop in human muscle and nervous tissue when eggs of *T. solium* are ingested.
Coenurus serialis	Sheep	*Taenia multiceps*	Dogs	*Coenurus serialis* develops in the brain and spinal cord of sheep, producing neurological symptoms.
Cysticercus bovis	Cattle	*Taenia saginata*	Humans	"Beef measles" • Humans become infected by ingesting *C. bovis* in under-cooked meat.
Hydatid cyst	Humans	*Echinococcus granulosus* and *E. multilocularis*	Dogs, cats	• Echinococcosis • Humans ingesting eggs of *E. granulosus* or *E. multilocularis* will develop hydatid cysts in the liver, lungs, brain, or other organs.

Trematodes

Like cestodes, trematodes (or flukes) are also flattened, but they are not segmented. Their shape is described as "leaf-like." Their eggs are capped, or operculated, and they are heavier than other parasite ova. The fecal sedimentation technique is used to isolate the heavy trematode eggs.

The life cycle of trematodes is more complex, involving many larval stages and at least one intermediate host. The definitive hosts are infected by ingesting the final larval stage.

Table 5.23   Trematodes of dogs and cats

Parasite	Definitive host(s)	Common name	Location of adult	Intermediate hosts	Distribution
Nanophyetus salmincola	Canine	Salmon poisoning fluke	Small intestine	1st: snail 2nd: salmon	Worldwide
Alaria spp.	Canine and feline	Intestinal fluke	Small intestine	1st: snail 2nd: frog, snake or mouse	Northern U.S. and Canada
Paragonimus kellicotti (Figure 5.26)	Canine and feline	Lung fluke	Lung parenchyma	1st: snail 2nd: crayfish	North America

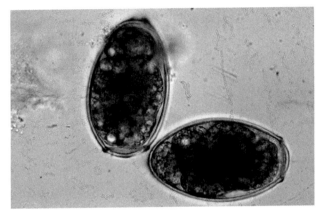

Figure 5.26   *Paragonimus kellicotti* (from Hendrix CM, Robinson E, *Diagnostic Parasitology for Veterinary Technicians*, 4th ed. St. Louis, MO: Mosby-Elsevier, 2012). *Source:* From Hendrix, Charles M, et al, (2012), ELSEVIER.

Table 5.24   Trematodes of ruminants

Parasite	Definitive host	Common name	Location of adult	Intermediate hosts	Distribution
Fasciola hepatica	Ruminants	Liver fluke	Bile duct	1st: aquatic snail 2nd: none, encysts onto aquatic vegetation	Worldwide

Protozoans

Protozoans are single-cell organisms which can infect a variety of body systems, such as the gastrointestinal tract and blood. In the trophozoite stage, the protozoa are capable of movement and reproduction. Transmission to a host typically occurs in the cyst stage of the protozoan life cycle.

Table 5.25   Gastrointestinal protozoans

Parasite	Definitive host(s)	Common name	Transmission route	Distribution	Testing method
Giardia spp. (Figure 5.17)	Dogs, cats, horses, ruminants, humans	Giardia	Ingestion of oocysts shed in the feces	Worldwide	Fecal flotation Direct smear (motile trophozoite can be occasionally observed) Immunological tests
Cystoisospora (Figure 5.27)	Dogs, cats, pigs	Coccidia	same as above	same as above	Fecal flotation
Eimeria leuckarti	Horses	Coccidia	same as above	same as above	Fecal flotation Fecal sedimentation
Eimeria bovis, Eimeria zuernii (Figure 5.28)	Ruminants	Coccidia	same as above	same as above	Fecal flotation
Toxoplasma gondii (Figure 5.27)	Feline (can infect humans)	Toxoplasma	same as above	same as above	Fecal flotation Immunological tests
Cryptosporidium spp. (Figure 5.29)	Dogs, cats, sheep, cattle, pigs, humans	Crypto	same as above	same as above	Fecal flotation
Tritrichomonas foetus (Figure 5.30)	Feline	Trichomonas	same as above	United States and United Kingdom	Fecal smear, fecal culture or PCR testing.

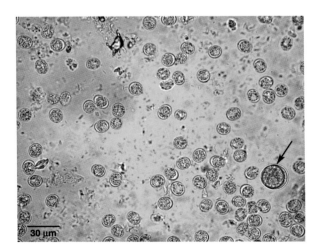

Figure 5.27   Small *Toxoplasma* oocysts. Also present is a larger *Isospora* oocyst (arrow). (From Zajac AM, Conboy GA, *Veterinary Clinical Parasitology*, 8th ed. Ames, IA: Blackwell Publishing, 2012). *Source:* From Zajac, Anne M. and Conboy, Gary A, (2012), John Wiley & Sons.

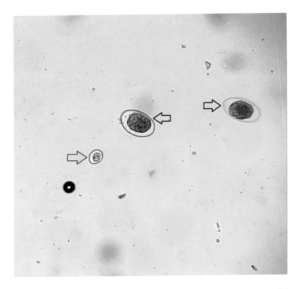

Figure 5.28 *Eimeria bovis* (red arrow) and *Trichostrongylus* spp. (black arrows) from a ruminant sample.

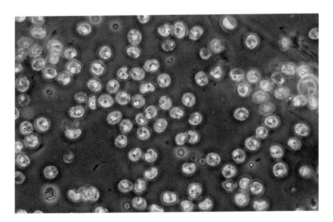

Figure 5.29 *Cryptosporidium* (from Hendrix CM, Robinson E, *Diagnostic Parasitology for Veterinary Technicians*, 4th ed. St. Louis, MO: Mosby-Elsevier, 2012). *Source:* From Hendrix, Charles M, et al, (2012), ELSEVIER.

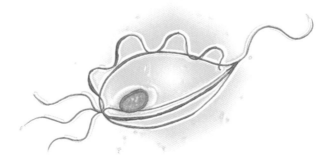

Figure 5.30 Diagram of *Tritrichomonas foetus*.

Table 5.26 Protozoans of the circulatory system

Parasite	Definitive host	Common name	Transmission route	Distribution	Testing method
Babesia canis (Figure 5.31)	Canine	Babesia	Bite of an intermediate host (tick)	Worldwide	Observation of organisms with the RBC on a stained blood smear Immunological testing
Babesia equi	Equine	Equine piroplasm	Bite of an infective tick	Worldwide	Observation of organisms with the RBC on a stained blood smear Immunological testing
Cytauxzoon	Feline	Cytauxzoon	Bite of an intermediate host (tick)	Africa and the U.S.	Observation of piroplasm inclusions in the RBCs on a stained blood smear
Hepatozoon canis and *Hepatozoon americanum*	Canine	Hepatozoon	Ingestion of an intermediate host (*Rhipicephalus sanguineus* for *H. canis* and *Amblyomma americanum* for *H. americanum*)	U.S., Asia, Europe, Africa	Observation of intracellular parasites in the leukocytes on a stained blood smear.

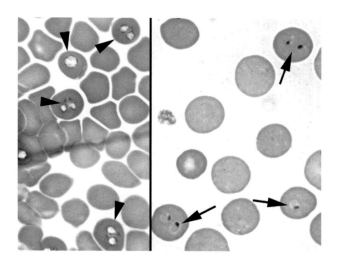

Figure 5.31 *Babesia canis* (left) and *Babesia gibsoni* (right) present on a canine blood film (from Thrall MA, Weiser G, Allison RW, Campbell TW, *Veterinary Hematology and Clinical Chemistry*, 2nd ed. Ames, IA: Blackwell Publishing, 2012). *Source:* From Thrall, Mary Anna, et al, (2012), John Wiley & Sons.

Table 5.27 Protozoans of the urogenital system

Parasite	Definitive host	Common name	Transmission route	Distribution	Testing method
Tritrichomonas foetus (Figure 5.30)	Bovine (reproductive tract)	Trichomonas	Sexual transmission	Worldwide	Examination of fluid collected from the stomach of an aborted fetus, vaginal and prepuce washings, or uterine discharge

Rickettsiae

Rickettsiae are intracellular, Gram-positive bacteria with a number of species which can infect the blood cells of its hosts. Rickettsiae are intracellular, Gram-positive bacteria with a number of species which can infect the blood cells of their hosts (e.g., *Anaplasma* spp.).

Table 5.28 Rickettsial parasites

Parasite	Hosts	Vector	Infected cells
Anaplasma spp.	Dogs, ruminants, horses	Ticks	Lymphocytes, platelets, or RBCs (species dependent)
Ehrlichia spp. (Figure 5.32)	Dogs, ruminants, horses	Ticks	Leukocytes, RBCs, and platelets (species dependent)

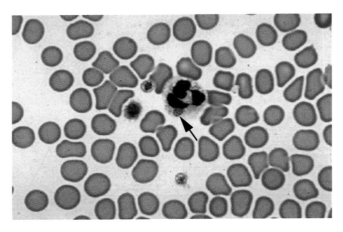

Figure 5.32 Peripheral blood film from a dog containing an *Ehrlichia ewingii* morula (arrow) in a neutrophil (from Thrall MA, Weiser G, Allison RW, Campbell TW, *Veterinary Hematology and Clinical Chemistry*, 2nd ed. Ames, IA: Blackwell Publishing, 2012). *Source:* From Thrall, Mary Anna, et al, (2012), John Wiley & Sons.

Common external parasites (ectoparasites) of domestic species

External parasites are arthropods, and only some are considered parasitic, while others may serve as an intermediate host or a vector of disease. Most external parasites are either insects (fleas and lice) or arachnids (mites and ticks). Insects possess 3 pairs of legs, 3 body sections (head, thorax, and abdomen), and antennae. Arachnids have 4 pairs of legs and 2 body sections (cephalothorax and abdomen) and do not possess antennae. Immature stages of both insects and arachnids differ in their appearance and anatomy.

Insecta

Lice

There are two types of lice: Mallophaga (biting lice) and Anoplura (sucking lice) (Table 5.29). Both are dorsoventrally flattened with no wings.

Lice can be collected using the cellophane tape technique or using a lice comb to collect the parasites onto a piece of paper. Due to their size, identification may be made without use of a microscope; however, examining under 40× magnification can be done to observe specific characteristics.

Table 5.29   Mallophaga (biting lice) and Anoplura (sucking lice)

Parasite	Hosts	Unique characteristics	Examples
Mallophagan species	Mammals and birds	Smaller of the two Usually yellow Large, rounded head	*Damalinia bovis* (cattle) *Trichodectes canis* (dogs) (Figure 5.33)
Anopluran species	Domestic mammals except cats. Not seen in birds	Larger than biting lice Grey, but can be red if they have consumed blood Narrow head	*Haematopinus suis* (pig) *Linognathus setosus* (dog) (Figure 5.34)

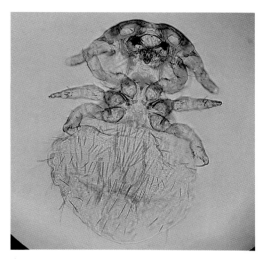

Figure 5.33   *Trichodectes canis* (chewing or biting louse).

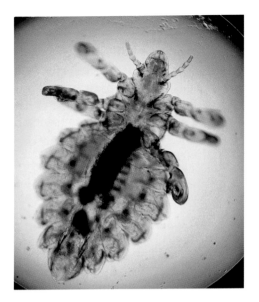

Figure 5.34 *Linognathus setosus* (sucking louse).

Fleas

Fleas (*Ctenocephalides* spp.) are small, wingless insects which have a laterally compressed body and strong hind legs used for jumping. Adult fleas suck blood from their hosts using siphon-like mouthparts. Females are typically larger than males (Figure 5.35). Fleas also serve as the intermediate host for *Dipylidium caninum* (tapeworm of dogs and cats).

Fleas can be difficult to collect due to their jumping ability. Using the cellophane tape technique on parted hair can be effective.

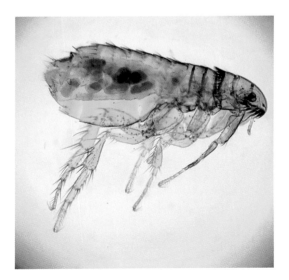

Figure 5.35 *Ctenocephalides* sp. (flea).

Diptera (two-winged flies)

Flies can contribute to disease in several ways. They can serve as vectors for disease or be a nuisance and affect efficiency of production animals (Table 5.30). Their larval stages produce a condition called myiasis, commonly referred to as maggots or fly strike, when the immature larval stage of the fly infects a host (Table 5.31). This can be facultative, meaning that the larvae can live on the host (i.e., fly strike), or obligatory, meaning that it is required that the larvae complete this stage of their life cycle within a host.

Table 5.30 Diptera (two-winged flies)

Fly	Host	Common name	Location
Melophagus ovinus (Figure 5.36)	Sheep and goats	Sheep ked	Skin surface, deep under the wool or fleece

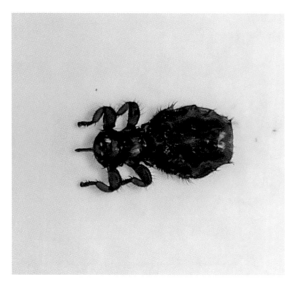

Figure 5.36 *Melophagus ovinus* (sheep ked).

Table 5.31 Myiasis-producing flies

Fly	Hosts	Common name	Location
Cuterebra spp. (Figure 5.37)	Rodents, occasionally dogs and cats	Warbles	Subcutaneous areas around the head and neck
Gasterophilus spp. (Figure 5.38)	Horses	Bot flies (adults) Horse bots (larvae)	Eggs are attached to leg hairs; 2nd- and 3rd-stage larvae attach to the gastric mucosa
Oestrus ovis	Sheep	Nasal bots	Nasal passages

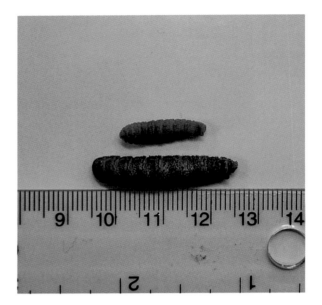

Figure 5.37 *Cuterebra* spp.

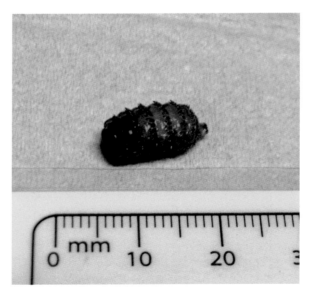

Figure 5.38 *Gasterophilus* sp. larva.

Acarina

Mites
Most parasitic mites spend their entire life cycle on their host and cause dermato-logic conditions referred to as mange.

Sarcoptiform mites are divided into two groups:
(1) Sarcoptidae (burrowing mites) (Table 5.32)
(2) Psoroptidae (nonburrowing mites) (Table 5.33)

Table 5.32 Sarcoptoidea (burrowing mites)

Parasite	Common name	Host(s)	Location of adult	Transmission	Description
Sarcoptes scabiei variety *canis* (Figure 5.39)	Scabies mite of dogs	Canine	Superficial layers of the epidermis	Direct contact	Oval Each leg possesses a "sucker" Terminal anal opening
Sarcoptes scabiei variety felis, suis, bovis, equi, and ovis	Scabies mite of cats, pigs, cattle, horses, and sheep, respectively	Cats, pigs, cattle, horses, and sheep, respectively	Superficial layers of the epidermis	Direct contact	As above
Notoedres cati	Feline scabies mite	Felines (occasionally rabbits)	Superficial layers of the epidermis Typically found around the ear pinna, face, neck, and feet	Direct contact	As above, except the anal opening is dorsal.

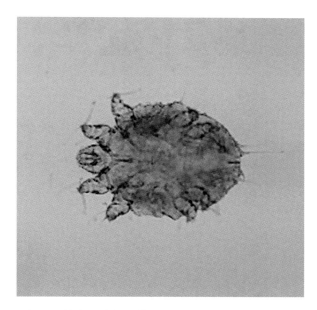

Figure 5.39 *Sarcoptes scabiei* (scabies mite).

Burrowing mites are collected using the skin scraping technique. Sampling should be done where the affected area meets the unaffected area.

Nonsarcoptiform mites include *Demodex* spp. (Table 5.34) and *Cheyletiella parasitivorax* (Table 5.35). *Demodex* spp. should be collected in the same manner as other burrowing mites.

Table 5.33 Psoroptidae (nonburrowing mites)

Parasite	Common name	Host	Location of adult	Transmission	Description
Psoroptes ovis, *Psoroptes bovis*, and *Psoroptes equi*	Scabies mite of sheep, cattle and horses, respectively	Sheep, cattle and horses, respectively	Skin surface on the body, withers and rump. Main and tail (*P. equi*)	Direct contact	Oval Possess a sucker at the end of some of their legs Adults possess 8 legs
Chorioptes equi, *Chorioptes bovis*, *Chorioptes caprae*, *Chorioptes ovis*	Foot and tail mite	Horses, cattle, goats and sheep, respectively	Surface of the skin, particularly on the shoulders, hind legs, and flanks.	Direct contact	Short pedicels with suckers on the end.
Otodectes cynotis (Figure 5.40)	Ear mite	Canine, feline and ferrets	External ear canal	Direct contact	Can be viewed as white motile objects with an otoscope Short pedicels with suckers on the ends of some legs Terminal anal opening

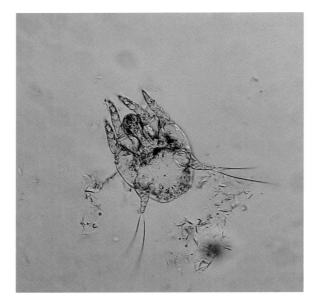

Figure 5.40 *Otodectes cynotis* (ear mite).

Table 5.34   Non-sarcoptiform mites

Parasite	Common name	Hosts	Location of adult	Transmission	Description
Demodex spp. (Figure 5.41)	Follicular mite, demodectic mange mite	Domestic animals and humans (host specific)	Hair follicles Sebaceous glands	Direct contact	Elongated, resembling alligators or cigars Short legs Adults have 8 legs, while larvae have 6

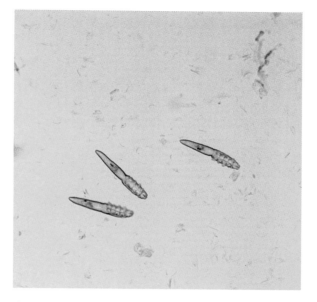

Figure 5.41   *Demodex* spp.

Table 5.35   Fur mites

Parasite	Common name	Hosts	Location of adult	Transmission	Description
Cheyletiella parasitovorax (Figure 5.42)	Walking dandruff	Dogs, cats, rabbits	Surface of the skin	Direct contact	Large mites (386 × 266 µm) Bell-pepper-shaped body Hook-like mouthparts

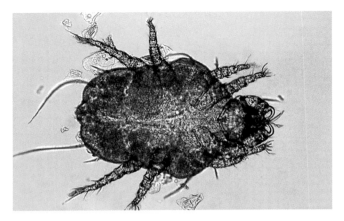

Figure 5.42 *Cheyletiella parasitovorax* (walking dandruff) (from Hendrix CM, Robinson E, *Diagnostic Parasitology for Veterinary Technicians*, 4th ed. St. Louis, MO: Mosby-Elsevier, 2012). *Source:* From Hendrix, Charles M, et al, (2012), ELSEVIER.

Ticks

Ticks are blood-sucking arachnids. They are dorsoventrally flattened and after feeding can become quite engorged and round (Table 5.36). Adults possess 8 legs; however, the nymph stage possesses 6. Ticks feed on a host and lay their eggs in the environment.

Hard ticks serve as vectors for a number of diseases, and some species produce a toxic saliva which causes tick paralysis in the host.

Table 5.36 Ticks

Tick species	Common name	Distribution	Disease vector
Ixodes scapularis (Figure 5.43)	Deer tick	Eastern U.S.	Tularemia *Babesia microti Borrelia burgdorferi* (Lyme disease) Tick paralysis
Rhipicephalus sanguineus (Figure 5.43)	Brown dog tick	North America	*Babesia canis*
Dermacentor variabilis (Figure 5.43)	American dog tick or wood tick	Eastern U.S.	Rocky Mountain spotted fever Tularemia
Dermacentor andersoni (Figure 5.44)	Rocky Mountain wood tick	Rocky Mountain regions	Rocky Mountain spotted fever
Amblyomma americanum (Figure 5.43)	Lone star tick	Southern U.S.; Midwest and Atlantic coast of the U.S.	Tularemia Rocky Mountain spotted fever

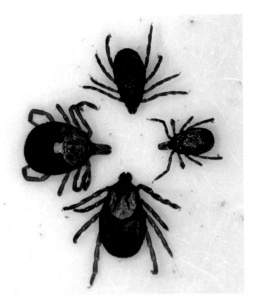

Figure 5.43 Female ticks of various species. (Right) *Ixodes scapularis* (deer tick); (bottom) *Dermacentor variabilis* (American dog tick); (left) *Amblyomma americanum* (Lone Star tick); (top) *Rhipicephalus sanguineus* (brown dog tick) (photo courtesy of Dr. Susan Little, Oklahoma State University, Stillwater, OK). *Source:* Courtesy of Dr. Susan Little, Oklahoma State University.

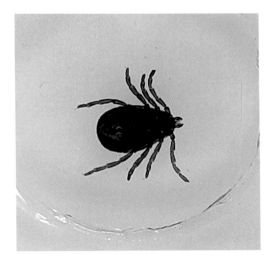

Figure 5.44 *Dermacentor andersoni* (Rocky Mountain wood tick).

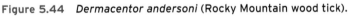

Zoonosis

There are a number of parasites encountered in veterinary medicine which pose a zoonotic risk (Table 5.37). Following proper safety protocols, including the use of appropriate personal protective equipment (PPE), and maintaining a high standard of cleanliness in the lab area can minimize the risk. Clients should be advised to speak with their primary health care provider should there be a concern regarding exposure to a zoonotic parasite.

Table 5.37 Parasites of zoonotic concern

Type	Parasite	Condition	Risk	Prevention
Nematodes	*Toxocara canis* and *Toxocara cati*	Visceral larva migrans (VLM) and ocular larva migrans (OLM)	• After ingestion of the parasite eggs, the larvae migrate through the tissues, organs and brain (VLM), causing disease in those systems. OLM occurs when the larvae migrate to the eye, causing vision impairment or blindness.	• Good hygiene practices when handling dog and cat feces. • Routine testing and administration of anthelmintics for dogs and cats.
	Ancylostoma caninum and *Uncinaria stenocephala*	Cutaneous larva migrans (CLM)	• Hookworm larvae present in the environment (typically sandy soil) penetrate exposed skin. • The larval activity causes migratory tracts, dermatitis and severe pruritus	• Routine testing and anthelmintics for pets • Protection of skin surfaces when visiting beaches where infected animals roam freely
	Trichinella spiralis	Trichinosis	• Humans become infected by eating pork infected with the larvae. • Symptoms include enteritis in the early stages. Later in the disease, larvae migrate throughout the body and encyst in the skeletal muscle causing vasculitis, muscle pain and weakness.	• Avoid consuming raw or undercooked meat. • Avoid consuming noninspected meat. • Wild game is another source of infection. • Freezing of meat can kill larvae.
Cestodes	*Taenia saginata*	Beef tapeworm	• Ingesting raw or undercooked beef which contains *Cysticercus bovis, the* metacestode stage of the tapeworm. Results in GI symptoms such as diarrhea, constipation or abdominal pain.	• Avoid consuming raw or undercooked meat. • Avoid consuming non-inspected meat.
	Taenia solium	Pork tapeworm	• Ingesting raw or undercooked pork which contains *Cysticercus cellulosae*, the metacestode stage of the tapeworm. • The embryo will hatch and migrate throughout the musculature, the subcutaneous tissues, and the brain and eye.	• Avoid consuming raw or undercooked meat. • Avoid consuming noninspected meat.

	Echinococcus granulosus and *Echinococcus multilocularis*	Hydatid disease	• After ingested eggs hatch, they travel to a variety of internal organs, including the brain, where they develop into cysts.	• Practicing good hygiene and hand washing. • Avoid feeding dogs raw livestock organ meat or allowing them to feed on wild rodents.
	Dipylidium caninum	Dipylidiasis	• Infection occurs most commonly in children when infected intermediate hosts (fleas) are ingested. • Symptoms include diarrhea, abdominal pain, and pruritus.	• Treat household pets for fleas; a flea control program should be implemented for all pets in the household.
Protozoans	*Toxoplasma gondii*	Toxoplasmosis	• May infect pregnant women, causing birth defect in the fetus • May infect immunocompromised individuals, causing seizures and vision and respiratory issues.	• Prevent fecal-oral transmission. • Wash hands after cleaning the litter box or encountering stray cats. Use of a mask is encouraged. • Do not consume undercooked meat.
	Cryptosporidium parvum	Cryptosporidiosis	• Produces transient, painful diarrhea when oocysts are ingested. • Chronic infections can last weeks to months.	• Wear gloves when gardening. • Using proper PPE and sanitation when handling young animals (especially calves) with suspected infections.
Arthropods	*Sarcoptes scabiei variety canis*	Canine scabies	• Humans become infected after coming into direct contact with an infested dog. • Pruritic skin lesions develop.	• Avoid contact with infested dogs. • Wear appropriate PPE if in contact with dogs with suspected infestations. • Treat infested dogs.

Chapter 6
Microbiology

Sample collection and handling

Various collection techniques can be employed to gather samples for microbiological evaluation. Regardless of the collection method, it is essential to follow strict aseptic techniques to avoid contamination and produce a diagnostic-quality specimen. If samples are not processed immediately, they should be preserved in a way that maintains the viability of the bacterial colonies.

Swab specimens

Rayon swabs are preferred over cotton for collection. The swab should be sterile and can be used to inoculate medium plates or prepare slides for staining. If the swab is to be sent to a reference lab, swabs which contain transport medium should be used for collection, as this will preserve the sample during shipping (e.g., Culturette) (Figure 6.1). It should be determined if the area to be cultured, and organism of interest, is of an aerobic or anaerobic nature in order to choose the correct swab and transport medium.

Fluid samples

Fluid samples (e.g., lung aspirates) should be collected using aseptic techniques and sterile equipment and stored in sterile containers. Red-top blood collection tubes work well for this purpose.

Urine samples

When a culture is desired, a urine sample should be collected by cystocentesis and stored aseptically. Sterile catheterization is an alternative. Voided samples should never be used, as contamination by normal flora and environmental bacteria is quite likely.

General guidelines for the shipping of samples

- Use transport medium (e.g., Culturette) to support the bacterial specimen during shipping.
- Refrigeration can extend the life of organisms. Do not allow the samples to freeze.

Veterinary Technician's Handbook of Laboratory Procedures, Second Edition. Brianne Bellwood and Melissa Andrasik-Catton.
© 2023 John Wiley & Sons, Inc. Published 2023 by John Wiley & Sons, Inc.
Companion website: www.wiley.com/go/bellwoodhandbook2

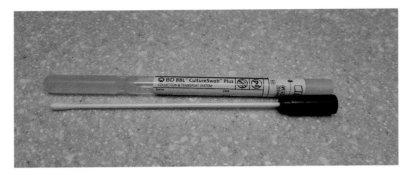

Figure 6.1   Collection swab with transport media.

- Ensure that all containers are well sealed and leakproof when shipping.
- Follow appropriate local guidelines for labeling and shipping of biological samples for transport.

Media and culture techniques

Culture medium is a material which supports the in vitro growth of microorganisms. Culture media can be liquid (e.g., broth) or solid (e.g., agar) and can also assist in identifying organisms through their selective and differentiating properties.

Enriched medium is a general-use medium with added nutrients and meets the growth requirements of most fastidious organisms (those with very specific and complex nutritional requirements). Added nutrients are in the form of blood, serum, or egg.
Selective medium supports the growth of certain microorganisms while inhibiting the growth of others. This will assist in isolating specific types of bacteria which may be difficult to isolate with other media, as they can become overwhelmed by the growth of other types of bacteria.
Differential medium contains an added indicator used to identify certain types of bacteria based on how they change that indicator (e.g., color change).
Slants are solid media contained within a tube. While setting, the tubes are held at an angle which allows the medium to solidify on a slant. This provides the opportunity either to culture organisms on the surface or to inoculate them deep into the medium.
Broths are liquid media which serve to cultivate and maintain profuse growth of microorganisms (e.g., bacteria and yeasts). They can be used for mixed bacterial cultures where the aerobic organisms will grow at the top of the broth and anaerobes will grow towards the bottom of the broth; however, the bacteria are not grown in individual colonies.

Common agar types

Trypticase soy agar
Trypticase soy agar (TSA) can also be referred to as a blood agar plate (BAP) (Figure 6.2). This is a general purpose nutrient medium used for culturing fastidious organisms and differentiating bacteria based on their hemolytic properties

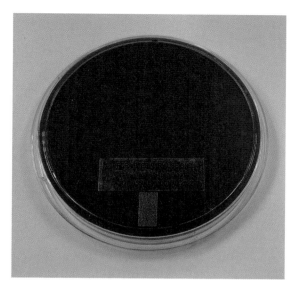

Figure 6.2 Trypticase soy agar (TSA) (Sensor Health Veterinary Diagnostics).

(e.g., *Streptococcus* spp.). This agar is classified as differential, as it displays 3 different types of hemolysis: alpha-, beta-, and gamma-hemolysis.

(1) Alpha-hemolysis: partial hemolysis that results in a green band or halo around the colonies.
(2) Beta-hemolysis: complete hemolysis that results in a clear zone surrounding the colonies.
(3) Gamma-hemolysis: no hemolysis around the colonies; the appearance of the agar remains unchanged.

MacConkey agar

MacConkey agar (MAC) is a selective and differential agar used for the growth of Gram-negative and enteric organisms (Figure 6.3). Crystal violet is added to suppress the growth of all Gram-positive organisms. It can also be classified as differential

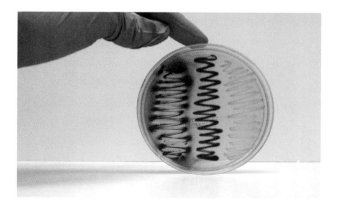

Figure 6.3 MacConkey agar (MAC). Lactose fermenters produce a pink color change (left), and non-lactose fermenters will not (right) (from Bassert JM, Beal AD, Samples OM, *McCurnin's Clinical Textbook for Veterinary Technicians,* 9th ed. St. Louis, MO: Elsevier, 2018). *Source:*From Hendrix, Bassert, Joanna M, et al, (2018), ELSEVIER.

and aid in bacterial identification, as it produces a color change to differentiate between lactose fermenters and non-lactose fermenters (e.g., *Escherichia coli*).

Mueller-Hinton agar

Mueller-Hinton agar (MH) is an enriched or general use media used with antimicrobial sensitivity testing, specifically disc diffusion or zone of inhibition testing (Figure 6.4).

Salmonella-Shigella *agar*

As with MAC, *Salmonella-Shigella* agar (SS) selects for Gram-negative bacteria and differentiates lactose fermenters and non-lactose fermenters. It can also differentiate H_2S-producing bacteria by developing a black color change in those colonies (e.g., *Salmonella* spp.).

Motility medium

Motility medium is a semisolid medium set in a tube which is used to detect the motility of microorganisms. A sample is inoculated deep into the medium using a straight wire, where color change occurs after bacterial growth (Figure 6.5). If the microorganisms are nonmotile, the color change will be limited to the stab track of the wire. If they are motile, the color change will diffuse beyond the track into the surrounding medium (e.g., *Proteus mirabilis*).

Combination plates

Combination plate agars are both selective and differential and used to identify certain bacterial species. The plates are split into quadrants with different chromogenic agars in each. Based on growth and color change, a species identification can be made using a reference guide (Figure 6.6).

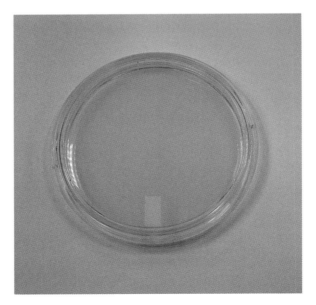

Figure 6.4   Mueller-Hinton (MH) agar (Sensor Health Veterinary Diagnostics).

(A)   (B)

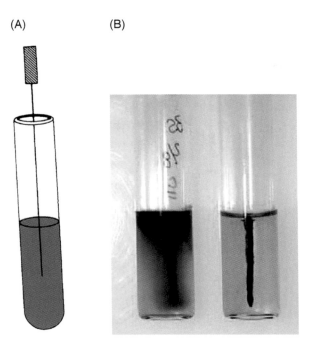

Figure 6.5   Motility media. (A) Inoculation of the tube is performed with a straight wire. (B) Motile growth (left) and nonmotile growth (right). (From Bassert JM, Beal AD, Samples OM, *McCurnin's Clinical Textbook for Veterinary Technicians,* 9th ed. St. Louis, MO: Elsevier, 2018). *Source:* From Hendrix, Bassert, Joanna M, et al, (2018), ELSEVIER.

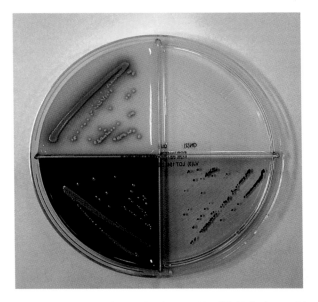

Figure 6.6   Combination plate (AgarSense by Sensor Health Veterinary Diagnostics).

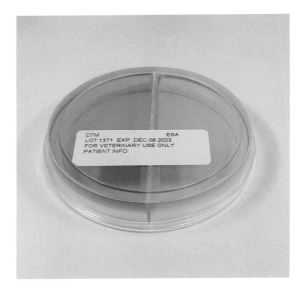

DTM
LOT 1371 EXP DEC.08.2022
FOR VETERINARY USE ONLY
PATIENT INFO:
ESA

Figure 6.7 Dermatophyte testing medium (DTM) on the left side of the plate and enhanced sporulation agar (ESA) on the right side. (DuoDermatophyte RW2 by Sensor Health Veterinary Diagnostics).

Dermatophyte testing medium

Dermatophyte testing medium (DTM) is used for the culturing of dermatophytes (e.g., *Trichophyton* spp.) and contains an antimicrobial agent to suppress the growth of bacteria. In the presence of most dermatophytes, the agar will turn red. DTM can often be found in a combination plate along with an agar which enhances the production of spores, which is useful for microscopic identification (i.e., enhanced sporulation agar [ESA]) (Figure 6.7).

Growth requirements

In addition to adequate nutrients, desirable environmental conditions must be provided to accommodate the growth requirements of different species of bacteria and fungi. Examples include oxygen requirements, humidity, and temperature, to name a few (Table 6.1). These can be achieved using incubators (Figure 6.8), gas packs, and anaerobic jars.

Table 6.1 Growth requirements

Group	Description
Obligate aerobes	Bacteria that require oxygen to survive
Obligate anaerobes	Bacteria that are killed in the presence of oxygen
Facultative anaerobes	Bacteria that can survive without oxygen; growth is limited.
Microaerophilic bacteria	Bacteria that require reduced levels of oxygen
Capnophilic bacteria	Bacteria that require high levels of carbon dioxide

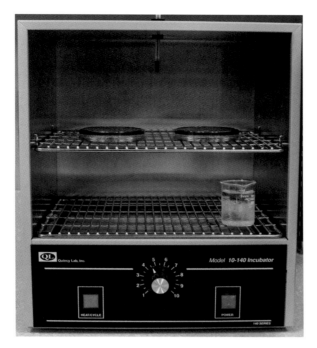

Figure 6.8   Compact in-house incubator. A container of water is added to provide humidity.

Staining

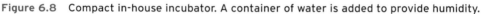

There are a number of different stains for bacteria and fungal organisms; however, the Gram stain and Ziehl-Neelsen (acid-fast) stain are the most common for bacteria. Lactophenol cotton blue is used to identify fungal organisms. More specialized stains are available to better visualize certain species or to visualize bacterial structures such as spores are flagella; however, they are not commonly used in veterinary practice.

Gram stain

The Gram stain set consists of a primary stain (crystal violet), a mordant (Gram iodine), a decolorizer (95% ethanol or acetone), and a counterstain (safranin) (Figure 6.9). The Gram stain procedure (Procedure 6.1) differentiates bacteria as Gram-positive or Gram-negative based on their cell wall structure. Visually, Gram-positive bacteria will appear purple, while Gram-negative bacteria will appear pink (Figure 6.10).

Procedure 6.1   Gram stain procedure

Materials
- Microscope slide
- Gram stain set
- Saline (optional)
- Flame or heat source
- Staining rack

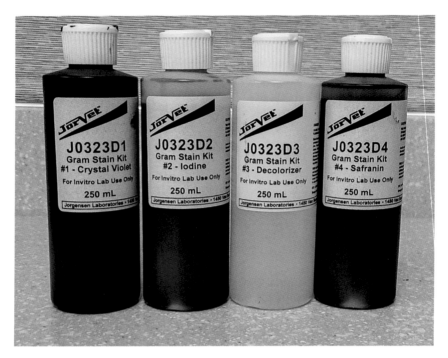

Figure 6.9   Gram stain kit.

Procedure

(1) Apply a thin layer of sample to a microscope slide. This is conducted with a sterilized microbiology loop to obtain a colony of bacteria from the culture medium. If the sample is too thick, mix a small amount into a drop of saline until it is homogenous.

(2) Allow the sample to fully dry.

(3) Heat-fix the sample by passing it over a flame 2 or 3 times (sample side up).

(4) Position the slide on a staining rack. Alternatively, an ice cube tray can be a substitute if a staining rack isn't available.

(5) Pour crystal violet over the sample and let sit for 1 minute.

(6) Rinse by dipping in tap water for 2 to 3 seconds.

(7) Pour iodine over the sample and let sit for 1 minute.

(8) Rinse by dipping in tap water for 2 to 3 seconds.

(9) Pour decolorizer over the sample and allow 15 seconds of contact.

(10) Rinse with tap water until no color appears.

(11) Pour safranin over the sample and let sit for 1 minute.

(12) Completely rinse with tap water.

(13) Allow to air dry. The slide may be blotted gently, but do not wipe.

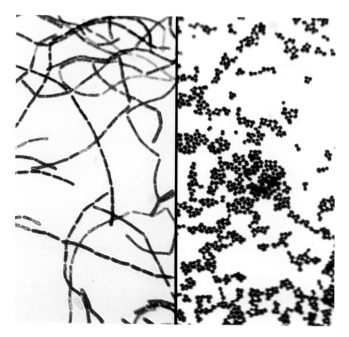

Figure 6.10 Gram-stained bacteria. Gram-negative bacteria appear pink (left), while Gram-positive bacteria appear purple (right).

Ziehl-Neelsen (acid-fast) stain procedure

Acid-fast stains (Procedure 6.2) are used to detect *Mycobacterium* and *Nocardia* species, which do not stain well with the Gram stain method. The oocysts of *Cryptosporidium* and *Isospora* from a cytology specimen (fecal smear) can also be identified with this stain. Visually, the organisms will appear bright red or pink against a green or blue background.

Procedure 6.2   Ziehl-Neelsen (Acid-Fast) stain procedure

Materials
- Microscope slide
- Flame or heat source
- Carbol fuchsin stain
- Acid alcohol decolorizer solution
- Malachite green or methylene blue
- Staining rack

Procedure
(1) Apply a thin layer of sample to a microscope slide and allow it to thoroughly air dry.
(2) Heat-fix the sample by passing it over a flame 2 or 3 times (sample side up).

(3) Flood the slide with carbol fuchsin stain and then heat the slide until the vapors rise

(4) Let cool for 5 minutes.

(5) Rinse with tap water.

(6) Rinse the slide with an acid alcohol solution for 60 seconds until it is decolorized.

(7) Rinse with tap water.

(8) Flood the slide with malachite green or methylene blue stain and let sit for 60 seconds.

(9) Rinse with tap water.

(10) Allow to air dry and examine microscopically.

Bacterial cell morphology

Shapes and arrangements

Upon microscopic examination, bacteria can be broadly classified by their shape (Table 6.2) and their color based on the Gram stain.

Gram staining can reveal either Gram-positive organisms (purple) or Gram-negative organisms (pink) (Figures 6.21 and 6.22). Comments regarding the arrangement of the bacteria can also be made, as different species may have characteristic growth patterns.

Other structures

Spores

Bacterial spores are a dormant stage which is highly resistant to environmental conditions, chemicals, and heat. They are formed under adverse conditions to support the viability of the bacteria until more favorable conditions return.

Spores can typically be seen microscopically as refractile bodies which resist Gram staining and can be located terminally, centrally, or subterminally on the bacteria. *Clostridium* spp. and *Bacillus* spp. are examples of species known to produce spores (Figure 6.23).

Bacterial spores are not reproductive as fungal spores are.

Capsules

Some species of bacteria are surrounded by a viscous substance called a capsule (e.g., *Pseudomonas aeruginosa*). Special staining methods are required to visualize these capsules microscopically. Capsules protect the bacteria from phagocytes, as they limit the phagocytes' ability to effectively engulf the microorganism. They also allow the bacteria to better adhere to surfaces, and their presence often correlates with the pathogenicity of the organism. Gram-negative bacteria are more likely to have a capsule (Figure 6.23).

Table 6.2   Bacterial shapes

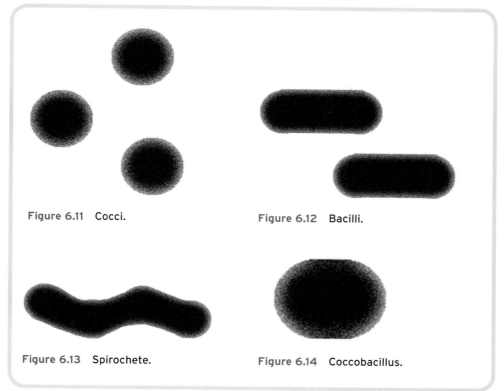

Figure 6.11   Cocci.

Figure 6.12   Bacilli.

Figure 6.13   Spirochete.

Figure 6.14   Coccobacillus.

Table 6.3   Bacterial arrangements

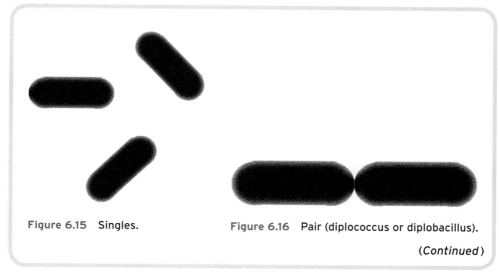

Figure 6.15   Singles.

Figure 6.16   Pair (diplococcus or diplobacillus).

(Continued)

Table 6.3 (*Continued*)

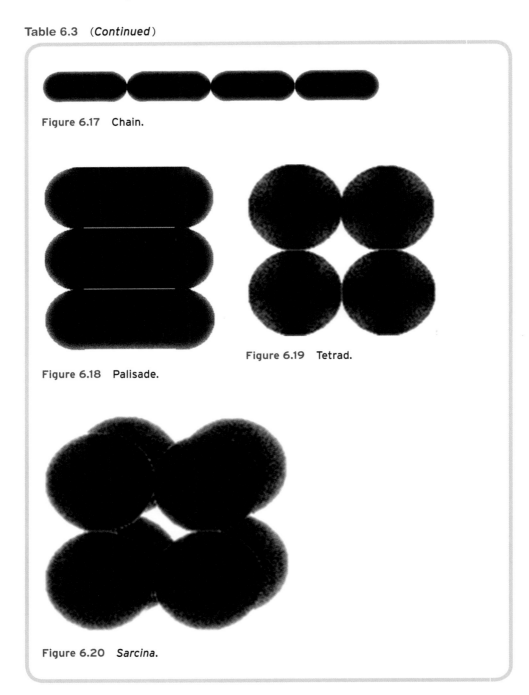

Figure 6.17   Chain.

Figure 6.18   Palisade.

Figure 6.19   Tetrad.

Figure 6.20   *Sarcina*.

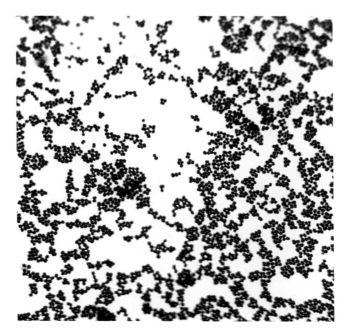

Figure 6.21 Gram-positive cocci in clusters (*Staphylococcus aureus*).

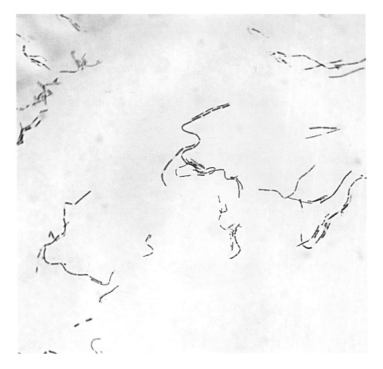

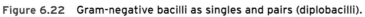

Figure 6.22 Gram-negative bacilli as singles and pairs (diplobacilli).

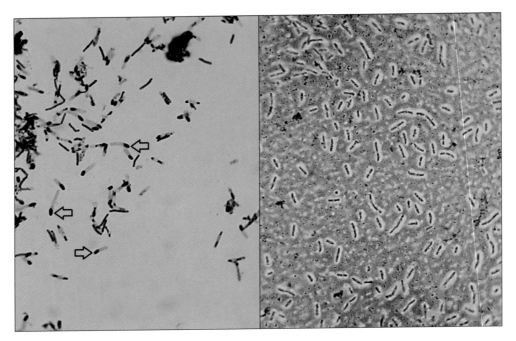

Figure 6.23 (Left) Gram-positive bacilli with spores (arrows). (Right) Capsules visualized with a capsule stain.

Flagella

Bacterial flagella are long, thin appendages that extend from the cell at either end or surround it completely. Flagella provide the bacteria with the ability to move and are found on some species (e.g., *Escherichia coli* and *Clostridioides difficile*). While the flagella are not visualized microscopically using standard Gram staining techniques, the motility of a bacterium can be assessed and the presence of flagella inferred.

Hanging drop testing for motility

The hanging drop method is one way to assess motility (Procedure 6.3). Bacteria are suspended in a liquid broth and are examined for movement. Another method for detecting motility is the use of motility media (see "Media and Culture Techniques," above).

Procedure 6.3 Hanging drop testing for motility

Materials
- Microscope slides with a depression
- Coverslip
- Petroleum jelly
- Wire loop
- Broth culture of bacteria

Procedure

(1) While holding a coverslip by the edges, apply a small amount of petroleum jelly to each corner.
(2) Collect a loop of fresh culture from the broth and add it to the center of the coverslip.
(3) Apply the microscope slide upside down over the coverslip so that the depression lines up with the drop of broth culture.
(4) Allow the petroleum jelly to adhere and seal the coverslip to the slide.
(5) Turn the slide over and allow the drop of broth culture to "hang" from the coverslip, suspended in the depression on the slide (Figure 6.24).
(6) Examine microscopically for motility.

It is important to differentiate Brownian movement from true motility. All organisms will display Brownian movement as they vibrate in a liquid suspension. True motility will appear as purposeful movement in a set direction.

Mycology

Several pathologic fungal organisms, as well as yeasts, are seen in veterinary medicine. One of the most common types of dermatophytes is known as ringworm, which are cutaneous fungal organisms. Common dermatophyte species include *Microsporum* spp. and *Trichophyton* spp.

Fungal organisms can be identified using culture medium kits or microscopic examination (Figure 6.25). Fungal organisms possess unique structures which can assist in identification. Hyphae are branch-like structures which can be cross-walled (septate hyphae) or nonseptate. Reproductive spores such as conidia or sporangiospores can also be visualized to assist in identification.

Yeasts do not produce reproductive spores; rather, they reproduce by budding (Figure 6.26).

Dermatophyte testing

When examining or collecting samples for dermatophyte testing, the areas around the periphery of the lesion should be sampled. Broken hair shafts and dry, flaky skin lesions should be collected, as they are most likely to harbor the organism.

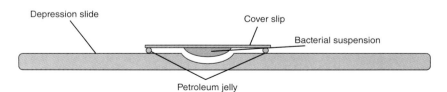

Figure 6.24 Hanging drop motility test.

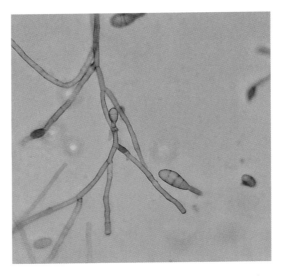

Figure 6.25 Fungal hyphae (septate) and spores (*Trichophyton* spp.).

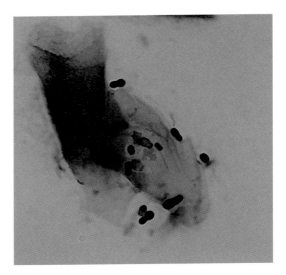

Figure 6.26 Budding yeast (*Malassezia pachydermatis*).

Direct exam

Hairs from an affected animal are collected and mounted in 10% potassium hydroxide (KOH). The slide is gently warmed and examined microscopically for the presence of spores on the hair shaft.

Alternatively, the cellophane tape prep technique can be used to collect surface debris; the tape is then mounted onto a microscope slide with an added drop of lactophenol cotton blue.

Wood's lamp

Some species of *Microsporum* spp. may fluoresce under a Wood's lamp; however, only 50% of cases will display the characteristic green fluorescence, and therefore, it is not reliable as the sole method for diagnosing dermatophytosis.

Culture

As mentioned above, DTM is used to culture dermatophyte organisms (Procedure 6.4). The agar will turn red in the presence of most dermatophytes, which can subsequently be examined microscopically for the presence of characteristic hyphae and spores (Figure 6.27).

Procedure 6.4   Dermatophyte collection and culture procedure

(1) Collect hair and skin samples from the periphery of the lesion using forceps or a toothbrush.
(2) Apply the sample to the surface of the DTM.
(3) Ensure that the sample is pressed firmly onto the surface of the media.
(4) Incubate upside down (lid on the bottom) at room temperature, in the dark, with the lid loosened so as to not cut off oxygen.
(5) Examine every 2 to 3 days for growth for a maximum of 10 days.

Results (Figure 6.27)
• DTM will turn from orange to red around the colonies
• ESA will turn from yellow to blue-green around the colonies
• Growth will appear white and fluffy or white with a granular texture.
• Some yeasts may also produce a color change; however, their colonies appear moist and bacterium-like, rather than fluffy like those of dermatophytes.

  Microscopic evaluation should follow all cultures; a wet mount should be prepared using lactophenol cotton blue. Clear cellophane tape can be used sticky side down to gently lift colonies from the medium and transfer them to a microscope slide (Figure 6.28).

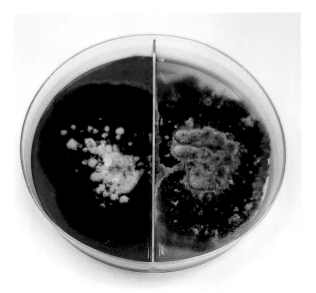

Figure 6.27   DTM/ESA test media displaying color change in the presence of dermophyte growth.

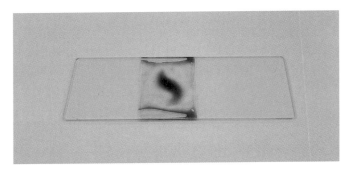

Figure 6.28 Wet mount prep for fungal examination using lactophenol cotton blue stain.

Yeasts

Microscopically, yeasts appear quite different from fungi. They are round and reproduce by budding. Examining for the characteristic budding or peanut-shaped organisms can aid in differentiating yeasts from other microscopic structures (Figure 6.29). Yeasts stain dark purple with Gram stain and Diff-Quik stain.

A commonly encountered yeast is *Malassezia pachydermatis*, which is a common cause of dermatitis and otitis externa.

Systemic dimorphic fungi

Dimorphic fungi appear similar to yeasts in their growth patterns and microscopic structures when growing in animal tissues. These fungal organisms are highly zoonotic and should be handled carefully (Table 6.4). Diagnosis can be made microscopically (Figure 6.30) or by serologic testing.

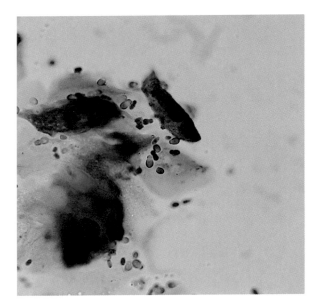

Figure 6.29 *Malassezia pachydermatis.*

Table 6.4 Dimorphic fungi of concern

Organism	Source	Geographical location	Hosts	Lesion location	Microscopic appearance
Blastomyces dermatitidis (Figure 6.30)	Acidic soil with high levels of organic material	Eastern North America	Dogs, cats, humans	Primary lesions in the lungs	Thick, double walled budding yeasts
Histoplasma capsulatum	Nitrogen rich soils; contamination with bat or bird droppings	Mississippi and Ohio river valleys	Dogs, cats, humans	Primary lesions in the lungs	Small yeasts with narrow attachments to mother cell
Coccidioides immitis	Desert soils	Semi-arid regions in southwest U.S., Central and South America	Dogs, cats, horses and humans	Primary lesions in the lungs	Spherules filled with endospores (in mature forms)
Sporothrix schenckii ("rose gardener's disease")	Old wooden posts, rose thorns, dead vegetation	Worldwide; more common in tropical areas (southern U.S.)	Dogs, cats, horses and humans	Subcutaneous nodules, lymphatic system	Elongated, cigar-shaped yeast appearance

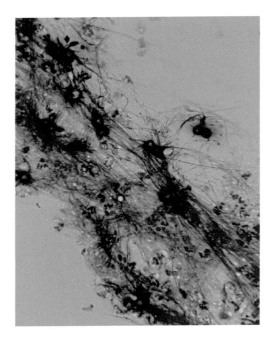

Figure 6.30   *Blastomyces* spp.

Chapter 7
Cytology

Cytology is a term that encompasses evaluation of cells from any place on or from within the body. It is typically an easy and fairly inexpensive method that can be used in the clinic to aid in diagnosis of parasitic diseases, infections, neoplasia, etc. Exfoliative cytology involves the examination of cells which have been collected off body surfaces or suspended in body fluids or secretions. By examining the cell types, cell numbers, and cell morphology and determining the presence of organisms, the technician can differentiate between an infectious, inflammatory, or neoplastic response. Due to the wide variety of sample types, the collection and preparation methods can vary significantly. Regardless of the sample type or technique, the goal is to obtain a sample with adequate cellular content to be of diagnostic value.

Sample collection methods

Swabs

Swabs are a useful collection method for sites which can be difficult to access by other methods. The objective is to collect the exfoliated superficial cells and examine microscopically for preliminary or diagnostic cytology (Procedure 7.1). These cells are delicate, and a gentle approach should be taken during collection to preserve their structure. Moistening the swab prior to collection can help to minimize cell damage. If a culture is required, sterile swabs and appropriate preservation media should be used. Examples of locations where this method is ideal are the ear canal, nasal cavity (Figure 7.1), fistulous tracts, and vaginal canal (see Figure 7.29).

Procedure 7.1   Swab collection method

Materials
- Cotton or rayon swabs
- 0.9% Saline
- Microscope slides
- Mineral oil (optional)

Veterinary Technician's Handbook of Laboratory Procedures, Second Edition. Brianne Bellwood and Melissa Andrasik-Catton.
© 2023 John Wiley & Sons, Inc. Published 2023 by John Wiley & Sons, Inc.
Companion website: www.wiley.com/go/bellwoodhandbook2

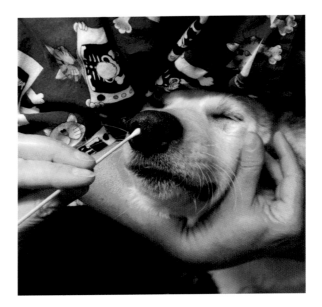

Figure 7.1 Swab collection of the nasal cavity.

Procedure

(1) Moisten the swab using 0.9% saline. Using an isotonic solution, such as saline, will allow the preservation of cellular integrity.

   If the sample will be used for culture, a sterile or commercial swab should be used.

(2) When culturing an infected area, the mucopurulent secretions should be avoided, as these contain high levels of contaminants which may obscure the desired cellular structures during examination.

(3) With appropriate restraint, insert the swab into the desired cavity and gently roll the swab against the mucosal surface or lining of the fistula, collecting the superficial cells. Avoid overly aggressive techniques such as twisting or scooping of the swab.

(4) To transfer the collected cells onto microscope slides, gently roll the swab along the length of the slide. Do not rub or "scribble" the swab onto the slide. Using a rolling technique will minimize cell damage (Figure 7.2).

(5) Allow slide to air dry and stain as desired.

Alternate method

(1) If the sample is to be examined for the presence of ear mites, mix the collected debris into a drop of mineral oil on the slide. Break up any large chunks of debris and examine for the presence of *Otodectes cynotis*.

The use of heat

In the case of ear swabs, there may be excessive wax present. Some individuals may apply *gentle* heat to degrade the wax; however, this is not a necessary step and can affect interpretation if done improperly. Applying a thin layer of the sample to the

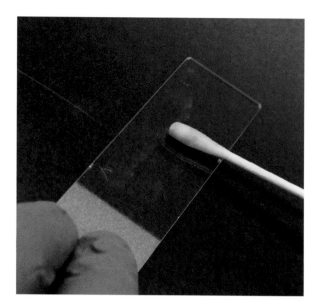

Figure 7.2 Rolling technique used to transfer collected material from the swab to the slide.

slide can also minimize the amount of wax. Heat is best applied using a hair dryer or a flame briefly directed to the underside of the slide. Excessive heat should be avoided, as it will damage the cellular structures. If a Gram stain is desired, the sample should be heat fixed according to the Gram stain procedure (see Procedure 6.1). Aside from these two scenarios, heat should never be applied to cytological samples.

Fine-needle biopsy

Fine-needle biopsies (FNBs) are used to collect cells from subcutaneous masses, lymph nodes, and organs. The advantage of this technique is that it avoids the superficial cells and other contaminants which may obscure the relevant cytological findings. Typically, the sample obtained contains a small number of cells with minimal amounts of blood and other fluids. Modifications to the technique are made to accommodate different types of masses in order to obtain the ideal sample.

Two variations of this technique include the aspiration and nonaspiration techniques (Figures 7.3 and 7.4). The nonaspiration technique is preferred in most instances, leading to less cellular damage and dilution of the sample due to blood contamination. When a mass is suspected to not be highly exfoliative (e.g., spindle cell-type masses), then the aspiration technique is appropriate.

Site preparation

In most cases, the site preparation for a FNB is no different from the preparation for a vaccination or venipuncture. Exceptions to this include a puncture into a body cavity or organ (e.g., joint cavity or liver) and situations in which a bacterial culture is to be performed, when surgical site preparation methods should be used.

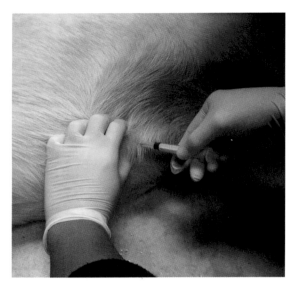

Figure 7.3   Fine-needle biopsy (aspiration technique).

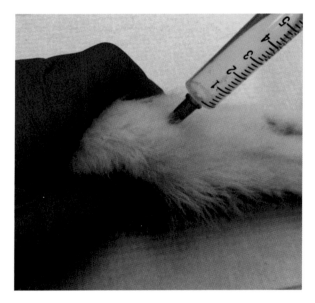

Figure 7.4   Fine-needle biopsy (nonaspiration technique).

Materials

Fine-needle biopsy sample collection requires the use of a needle (to penetrate the mass) and a syringe (to provide suction in the aspiration technique) (Procedures 7.2 and 7.3). The needle sizes used range from 21 gauge to 25 gauge, and the syringe size varies from 3 mL to 12 mL. The goal of the collection is to obtain representative, individual cells with minimal blood contamination or cellular damage. Adjusting the sizes of the needles and syringes will allow flexibility between masses of different firmness.

A softer mass requires a smaller needle and syringe to minimize blood or fluid contamination, whereas a firmer mass requires needles and syringes on the large end of the range, as these types of masses do not exfoliate as well and require more negative pressure from the syringe. Using an overly large needle would result in a core tissue sample, rather than individual cells. It will also produce other undesirable outcomes, such as blood contamination and excessive tissue trauma. One final consideration is the comfort of the technician collecting the sample. The syringe will need to be manipulated with one hand; therefore, one should take note of what size syringe would be comfortable to properly handle.

Procedure 7.2   Fine-needle biopsy (aspiration technique)

Materials
- Microscope slides
- Surgical prep materials (if required)
- 21-gauge to 25-gauge needle
- 3- to 12-cc syringe

Procedure
(1) With one hand, stabilize the mass.
(2) Insert the needle into the mass.
(3) Retract the plunger of the syringe, only once, and hold to create negative pressure (Figure 7.3).
   Prolonged aspiration or repeated pulses of negative pressure can damage cells and encourage blood contamination.
(4) While maintaining negative pressure and without exiting the mass, redirect the needle several times. This may be possible only with larger masses, and redirecting is not done for body cavities or organs. Sampling from undesirable areas surrounding the mass should be avoided. There should be no visible material within the syringe hub during this procedure.
(5) Release the plunger of the syringe.
(6) Exit the mass.

Procedure 7.3   Fine-needle biopsy (nonaspiration technique)

Materials
- Microscope slides
- Surgical prep materials (if required)
- 21-gauge to 25-gauge needle
- 3- to 12-cc syringe (if desired)

Procedure
(1) With one hand, stabilize the mass.
(2) Insert the needle into the mass.
   - A needle is used without a syringe attached.
   - If desired, a syringe can be used for easier handling, but negative pressure is never applied. The syringe should have a small amount of air aspirated into it prior to inserting into the mass.

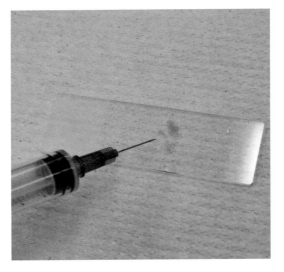

Figure 7.5 Expelling aspirated material onto the slide.

(3) The needle is moved in a stabbing motion redirecting within the mass.
(4) Exit the mass.

Transferring the sample to a slide (both techniques)

(1) Remove the needle from the syringe (if a syringe was used) and fill the syringe with air.
(2) In a quick motion, expel the components onto the center of a microscope slide.
(3) This expulsion of contents can be attempted multiple times until all cells from the needle have been expelled; however the syringe should be removed and reattached each time it is reloaded with air (Figure 7.5).
(4) Smear the sample using the desired method (a proper squash prep method is preferred). The sample will air dry quickly; therefore, slide preparation should be performed immediately.
(5) When dry, stain as desired.

Tissue biopsy (punch/wedge)

A tissue biopsy involves sampling a small section of tissue, rather than individual cells, and requires sedation or local/general anesthesia to perform. Once collected, the sample is useful for cytological or histological examination. Sites biopsied include superficial locations, such as skin or masses, internal organs (using ultrasound-guided biopsy techniques), and intestine (using an endoscope).

Site preparation depends on the sample to be collected. A surgical prep is required when a body cavity will be penetrated in order to biopsy an organ. Skin biopsy locations are prepped only by clipping the surrounding hair. Scrubbing the area or removing any superficial debris is not recommended.

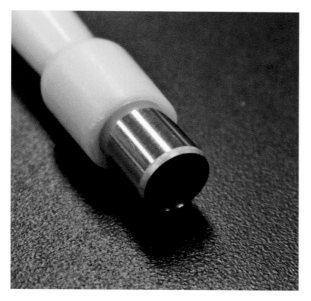

Figure 7.6 Punch biopsy with circular cutting blade.

Tissue biopsy—punch

A circular biopsy punch allows a representative sample which extends through multiple layers of tissue to be obtained quickly (Figure 7.6). Using slight downward pressure and rotation, the punch cuts through the tissue (Procedure 7.4). Various sizes of biopsy punches are available and typically range from 3 mm to 8 mm in diameter.

Procedure 7.4 Punch biopsy procedure

Materials
- Biopsy punch of desired size
- Thumb forceps
- Tissue scissors

Procedure
(1) Place the biopsy punch, blade side down, onto the surface of the sampling site.
(2) Gently rotate the punch in one direction until the tissue layer has been sectioned.
(3) Remove the punch.
(4) Gently grasp the edge of the sample with fine-toothed tissue forceps.
(5) Trim any subcutaneous tissue attached to the biopsy sample with tissue scissors or a scalpel blade.
(6) After collection, fresh impression smears can be made if appropriate.
(7) For histological evaluation, smaller samples can be allowed to dry onto a wooden tongue depressor, which serves as a splint. Once dry, the specimen and the splint should be submerged in 10% neutral buffered formalin.

Tissue biopsy—wedge

Wedge biopsy samples are collected using a scalpel blade to excise a small piece of tissue, often from a larger, surgically removed mass. When selecting the tissue to excise, be sure the sample contains tissue from the lesion, the transition zone, and normal tissue. This will allow the pathologist to examine the microscopic features as they transition from normal to abnormal. Once collected, the sample is processed in the same manner as in the punch method.

Impression smears

Impression smears, or imprints, can be made to collect samples from superficial lesions and surfaces or from biopsy samples (Procedures 7.5 and 7.6). Superficial cells are transferred onto a slide with little cellular disruption; however, only the superficial cells are collected using this technique. These cells may not be representative of the entire lesion and may represent only a secondary bacterial infection or inflammatory response. With biopsy samples or larger masses, the mass can be cut in half and imprints are made of the cross-section of tissue (Procedure 7.7).

Procedure 7.5   Impression technique for external lesions

Materials
- Microscope slides
- Gauze

Procedure
(1) For external lesions, little preparation is required. Any fluid or blood should be dabbed off with gauze prior to sampling.
(2) Place a slide face down onto the lesion and press. Do not rub or scrape the slide across the lesion.
(3) Lift the slide off and air dry before staining.

Procedure 7.6   Tzanck technique for external lesions

Materials
- Microscope slides (minimum of 5)
- Saline
- Gauze

Procedure
(1) Imprint with no cleaning or prep of the lesion.
(2) Clean the lesion with saline, then imprint again.
(3) Debride the lesion and imprint again.
(4) If present, imprint the underside of the scab that was debrided.
(5) Imprint the fresh tissue exposed after scab removal multiple times.

Procedure 7.7   Impression technique for tissue biopsies

Materials
- Tissue biopsy
- Forceps
- Gauze
- Microscope slides

Procedure
(1) A representative sample of the mass or lesion collected should be gently handled using forceps. Any excess blood can be gently dabbed off with gauze.
(2) Gently dab the sample several times along the length of your slide, making many impressions. Do not rub or scrape the tissue along the slide (Figure 7.7).
(3) If the sample is large, continue onto another slide to create more impressions.
(4) Allow slides to air dry before staining.

Scrapings

Scrapings are indicated for areas of flat skin or on tissues which exfoliate poorly. The sample will yield superficial cells only, which may not always be indicative of the lesion itself and could represent a secondary infection or inflammation. This technique is also commonly used to identify *Demodex* spp., the burrowing mite responsible for demodicosis, and other mite species (Procedure 7.8).

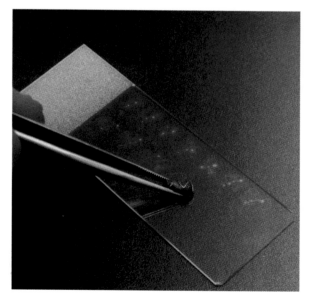

Figure 7.7   Imprints of biopsied tissue.

Procedure 7.8   Skin scraping collection technique

Materials
- No. 10 scalpel blade
- Microscope slides
- Mineral oil (optional)

Procedure
(1) Choose an area of hair loss or gently clip the location for scraping. Squeeze and roll this location between your fingers to open the hair follicles.
(2) Apply a coating of mineral oil onto the blade prior to scraping if examining for parasites. Do not use oil if planning a cytological examination.
(3) Anchor the skin with one hand for stability. Stretch the skin to remove any folds.
(4) Hold the scalpel blade perpendicular to the skin surface (Figure 7.8).
(5) Scrape the blade by pulling horizontally several times. A build-up of cells begins to develop on the edge of the blade.
(6) Spread the sample onto a slide.
 - For cytological examination, use the compression technique to gently make a smear. Allow to air dry and stain.
 - To examine for parasites, mix the sample into a drop of mineral oil on the slide and use the scalpel blade to thin the sample.

Centesis

A centesis is a puncture into a body cavity, using a needle, to obtain a sample of the fluid present within that cavity (Table 7.1).

Before collection, a surgical preparation should be performed. Restraint techniques range from physical restraint to general anesthesia, depending on the collection site. Once collected, the fluid is examined grossly and microscopically (Procedure 7.9).

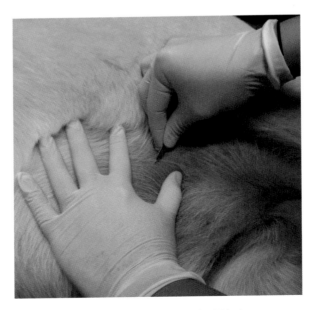

Figure 7.8   Skin scraping technique using a no. 10 scalpel blade.

Table 7.1 Common fluid samples

Sample type	Collection method
Abdominal fluid	Abdominocentesis or paracentesis
Thoracic fluid	Thoracocentesis or thoracentesis
Urine	Cystocentesis
Joint fluid	Arthrocentesis
Cerebrospinal fluid (CSF)	Cisternal puncture or lumbar puncture

Fluid may be centrifuged to concentrate the cells for slide preparation or placed into plain and/or anticoagulant collection tubes for further diagnostics.

Procedure 7.9   Centesis collection

Materials
- Needle, butterfly catheter, or indwelling catheter
- Surgical prep materials
- 6- to 60-cc syringe
- Microscope slides
- Ethylenediaminetetraacetic acid (EDTA) collection tubes and plain red-top tubes

Important points
- The gauge of needle or butterfly catheter will vary with the sample collection site and the patient being sampled.
- A safe way to withdraw large amounts of fluid is to use an indwelling catheter. The catheter is inserted into the cavity and needle removed. A syringe is attached and fluid is drawn out.
- Smears should be made immediately after fluid is collected, and any remaining fluid should be placed in EDTA and plain red-top tubes.
- A visual examination of the fluid should be made, noting color, turbidity, and volume collected.
- A total protein or specific gravity test should be performed on the fluid.
- During slide evaluation, total nucleated cell counts, types, and morphological assessments should be performed.
- In samples with low cellularity, a portion of the collected fluid can be centrifuged to concentrate the cellular components. After centrifugation, the sediment is examined microscopically. The remaining, unspun sample should be saved for other methods of analysis.

Fluid sample preparation techniques

Due to variation in the consistency of cytology samples, there are several different methods available to prepare a smear. The method should be chosen with consideration of the thickness of the sample and the planned evaluation and staining procedure to follow. Whenever possible, multiple smears should be prepared and evaluated for quality.

Bullet smear/blood smear technique

The bullet smear technique is performed in the same manner as the blood smear technique (Procedure 2.1 and Figure 2.1) and is useful with fluid samples which are highly cellular. Cells are spread thinly, and their morphology can be easily assessed.

Line smear technique

The line smear is designed to concentrate cells in a small area on the slide and is useful in fluid samples with low cellularity (Procedure 7.10). The disadvantage of this technique is that the cells are not spread flat, and detailed morphology of the cytoplasm and inclusions may be difficult.

Procedure 7.10 Line smear technique

(1) Add a drop of sample to one end of the slide.
(2) Using a spreader slide at an angle of 30°, back up into the drop and allow it to spread horizontally.
(3) Push the spreader slide forward while maintaining a consistent angle and contact with the base slide.
(4) Stop before creating a feathered edge, typically ¾ of the smear, and lift the spreader slide straight up and off the base slide (Figure 7.9).
(5) This will leave a concentrated line of sample, where examination of cells can take place.
(6) Allow to air dry.

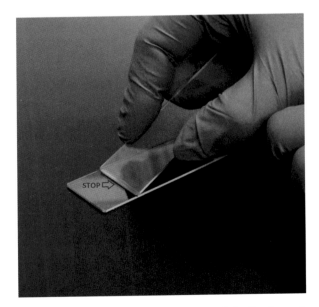

Figure 7.9 Line smear technique. Back the spreader slide into the drop of sample. When moving forward, stop before creating a feathered edge.

Centrifugation concentration

An alternative approach to samples with low cellularity is to concentrate the sample through centrifugation prior to making a smear (Procedure 7.11). Care should be taken not to cause damage to the cells during this process.

Procedure 7.11   Centrifugation concentration

(1) Centrifuge the sample at 1000 rpm to 1500 rpm for 5 minutes.
(2) Gently remove most of the supernatant while taking care not to disturb the sediment.
(3) Resuspend the sediment with a couple of drops of supernatant by tapping the side of the tube.
(4) Prepare a smear using the bullet, line smear, or compression technique.

Tissue sample preparation techniques

Compression technique/squash prep technique

Samples collected from tissue masses do not spread as easily as fluid samples. Because of this, the smear preparation methods discussed above are not useful. The compression technique works well for thicker samples (Procedure 7.12). Care must be taken to avoid the rupturing of cells with this technique.

Procedure 7.12   Compression technique/squash prep technique

(1) After adding your sample to the center of a base slide, place another spreader slide over top of the base slide at a 90° angle (Figure 7.10).

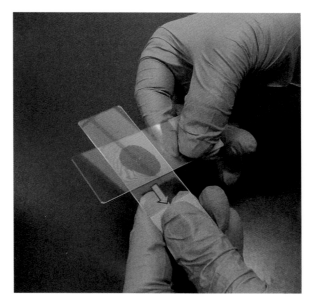

Figure 7.10   Compression smear technique.

(2) Allow the weight of the slide to "squash" the sample. Do not apply any additional pressure as this could damage the cells.
(3) Slide the spreader slide off the base slide to spread the sample out. Avoid any downward pressure while performing this.
(4) Allow to air dry.

Modified compression technique

This technique is similar to the compression technique; however, it is slightly gentler on cells and is useful if the compression technique results in cell rupture (Procedure 7.13).

Procedure 7.13   Modified compression technique

(1) After adding your sample to the center of a base slide, place another spreader slide over top of the base slide.
(2) Allow the weight of the slide to squash the sample.
(3) Instead of sliding the spreader slide, rotate it so that it is angled at the other end of the slide (Figure 7.11).
(4) Lift the spreader slide upward to reveal the smear.
(5) Allow to air dry.

Starfish technique

The starfish technique is another option for fragile cells (Procedure 7.14). The disadvantage is that the sample will remain thick, which can affect the accuracy of the morphological examination.

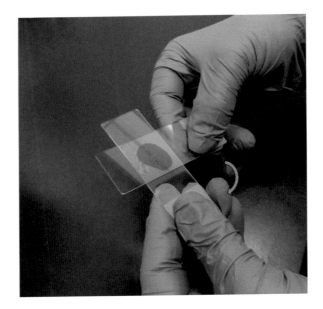

Figure 7.11   Modified compression technique.

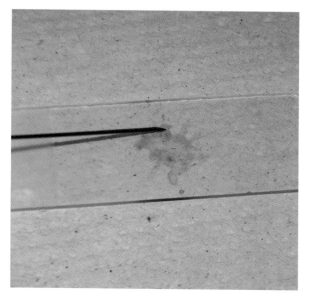

Figure 7.12   Starfish technique.

Procedure 7.14   Starfish technique

(1) After the sample has been added to the slide, use a needle to drag the sample outward in multiple directions to thin it (Figure 7.12).
(2) Allow to thoroughly air dry, as this is a thicker prep.

Staining techniques

Romanowsky stains

There are several types of stains used for cytology examination. Romanowsky-type stains (e.g., Diff-Quik and Wright's) are commonly found in veterinary hospitals and result in adequate cellular detail (Figure 7.13). Some mast cell granules will not stain with Diff-Quik. This may be corrected by increasing the fixation time to 15 minutes. Smears should be allowed to air dry prior to staining (see Procedure 2.2 for the Diff-Quik staining method).

When staining, the thickness of the sample should be taken into consideration. Thicker samples should be exposed to the staining solutions for longer periods of time, whereas thinner samples will stain better with shorter exposure to the stain.

The lab should maintain a set of stains for "clean" cytology (e.g., lymph node aspirates and joint fluid samples) and "dirty" cytology (e.g., ear swabs and purulent draining tracts).

New methylene blue stain

New methylene blue (NMB) provides excellent nuclear detail; however, it stains the cytoplasm quite poorly (Figure 7.14). This can be an advantage with high numbers of red blood cells in the sample, as they will stain pale and not obscure any nucleated cells.

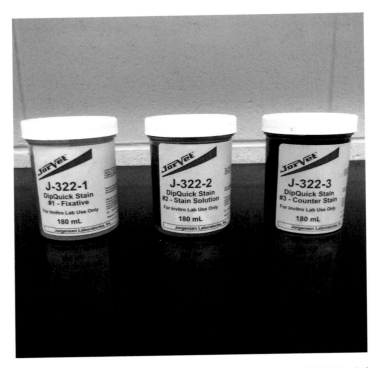

Figure 7.13 DipQuick stain set. A set of "clean" stains and a set of "dirty" stains should be available to use for different cytology samples. *Source*: Jorgensen Labs

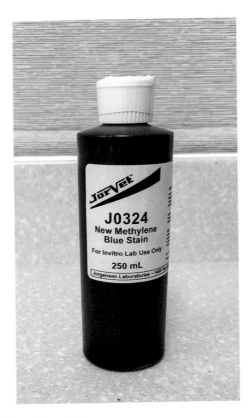

Figure 7.14 New methylene blue stain.

Papanicolaou stains

Papanicolaou stains provide excellent nuclear and cytoplasmic detail. The staining procedure requires multiple steps, is time consuming and the solutions can be difficult to acquire. The smears must be wet fixed, before the sample has dried to the slide. For these reasons, Papanicolaou staining isn't practical for most veterinary hospitals.

Gram staining

A Gram stain can be useful when evaluating bacterial pathogens within the sample. Cellular staining is not adequate for cytological assessment; however, bacterial morphology can aid in diagnosis (see Procedure 6.1 for the Gram stain method).

General tips for submitting cytology slides and tissue samples to the laboratory

- Provide a detailed patient history pertaining to the lesion (duration of problem, growth rate, whether the animal exhibits pruritus or pain, etc.).
- Comment on the physical appearance of the lesion. Is it a tumor, nodule, or cyst? Is there alopecia, hyperpigmentation, etc.?
- Describe the location of the lesion or mark the location on a diagram. If a representative sample of a larger lesion is being sent, indicate the size of the original lesion.
- Prepare multiple slides and submit both air-dried and Romanowsky-stained smears.
- If submitting fluid samples, prepare fresh smears to send along with the fluid.
- Label the smears clearly, noting the sample collection source for each smear. (e.g., if submitting multiple lymph node FNBs, note which slides correspond to which lymph node).
- Protect the slides from breakage during shipment using slide mailers.
- Tissue samples should be preserved in formalin prior to shipping. In northern climates, formalin may freeze during shipping in the winter months. Reference laboratories may recommend that a specimen be fixed in formalin for 24 hours and then shipped in alcohol. This procedure should be confirmed with the lab prior to shipment, and it should be indicated on the requisition form.
- Do not package unfixed slides with any samples that contain formalin. Formalin fumes will interfere with the staining results of slides that are exposed.
- Ensure that all slides and containers are fully labeled with patient information, date, and sample type.

If cytology slides are to be sent to the reference laboratory, at minimum, the following assessments should be made microscopically prior to shipment:

Is the sample adequately cellular?
- Ensure that there are in fact cells present for the pathologist to examine. If not, consider a concentration technique, such as a line smear or centrifugation of the fluid.

Is the sample what was expected?
- Examine any FNB collections for expected cell types to ensure that the target was not missed.

Are the cells intact?
- Even a very cellular sample is unusable if the cells are all ruptured. Prepare new slides using a less traumatic smear technique.

Fluid cytology assessment

Gross sample description

When fluid samples are analyzed, several initial physical assessments are made on the fluid itself prior to the microscopic exam. These include assessing the color, odor, and turbidity. Protein levels and a total nucleated cell count (TNCC) are also measured. Automated analyzers may be able to analyze the fluid cytology and produce a TNCC. These assessments should be performed on fluid collected in EDTA tubes.

While variations exist between different fluid types, there are consistent trends with changes in color, clarity, protein, and TNCC when normal samples are compared to inflammatory samples.

Respiratory samples

A transtracheal wash is used to collect samples from the trachea and bronchi. To collect samples from the nasal cavity, a nasal flush is used (Table 7.2). Once collected, the sample may need to be centrifuged if it has low cellularity.

Pleural and peritoneal fluid

The appearances of normal fluids from the pleural and peritoneal cavities have similar characteristics (Table 7.3). Exudative fluids have increased TNCCs and protein levels due to inflammation. Further microscopic evaluation of the inflammatory cells present can help to classify the inflammation. Transudative fluids are noninflammatory and therefore do not possess the increase in turbidity and TNCC seen in the exudative samples. Hypoproteinemia is an example of a transudative

Table 7.2 Normal microscopic appearance of a transtracheal wash sample

Feature	Comments
TNCC	Not typically assessed; variable and subjective
Normal cell types	Columnar epithelial cells
	Cuboidal epithelial cells
	Neutrophils
	Macrophages
Inflammatory changes	Increased TNCC
	Increased neutrophils and macrophages
	Increased amount of mucus
Allergy-induced changes	Eosinophils present
Pathogens	Bacteria, fungi

Table 7.3 Properties of pleural and peritoneal fluid samples

Sample type	Color	Turbidity	Protein concn (g/dL)	TNCC	Cell types
Normal	Colorless to straw yellow	Clear to slightly cloudy	<2.5	2000–6000 cells/μL	• Macrophages, lymphocytes, mesothelial cells • Minimal erythrocytes
Exudate	White or pale yellow	Turbid	>2.5	Increased >5000 cells/μL	Inflammatory cells • Neutrophils (may be degenerate or nondegenerate) • Macrophages (Figure 7.16) • Possibly lymphocytes and eosinophils • Septic effusions will have phagocytosed microorganisms (typically bacteria) and increased amounts of degenerate neutrophils (Figure 7.20)
Transudates	Colorless	Clear	<2.5	<1500 cells/μL	Macrophages, lymphocytes, mesothelial cells, nondegenerate neutrophils
Modified transudates	Typically clear	Slightly cloudy	2.5–5.0	1000–5000 cells/μL	• Lymphocytes and macrophages • Low numbers of nondegenerate neutrophils and mesothelial cells

effusion. Modified transudates are a result of fluid leakage from the lymphatic vessels. Because this fluid also contains proteins and potentially cellular elements, the term "modified" is used to differentiate this type from transudates. Congestive heart failure is a common cause of modified transudative effusion.

Synovial fluid

Normal synovial fluid samples provide a very small sample, often only one or two drops. This can limit the number of evaluations made on the fluid. In cases of inflammation or degenerative arthropathy, the volume may be increased. In addition to the gross examination and more specific cell counts, the viscosity of synovial fluid should also be assessed (Table 7.4).

Table 7.4 Properties of synovial fluid samples

Sample type	Color	Turbidity	Protein concn (g/dL)	TNCC (cells/μL)	Cell types	Viscosity
Normal	Colorless to pale yellow	Clear	<2.5	<3000 (dogs) <1000 (cats)	• Lymphocytes, monocytes and macrophages • Few neutrophils	High (>2-cm string)
Degenerative arthropathy	Colorless	Clear	Mild increase (<4.0)	1000–10,000	• Lymphocytes, monocytes and macrophages • Few neutrophils	Decreased depending on severity
Arthritis	Yellow-white	Cloudy	>3.0	4000–>10,000	• Large amounts of neutrophils • Small numbers of mononuclear cells	Decreased depending on severity
Hemarthrosis	Orange-red	Cloudy	Increased	3000–5000	• Erythrocytes • Lymphocytes, monocytes and macrophages • Few neutrophils	Decreased

Table 7.5 Normal CSF properties

Color	Colorless
Turbidity	Clear
Protein	0.05 g/dL
TNCC	<25 cells/μL
Cell types seen	Mononuclear cells (generally lymphocytes)

The viscosity of the fluid correlates to the quality of hyaluronic acid and lubrication properties of the synovial fluid. Normal fluid is sticky, and viscosity can be assessed by placing a drop between two fingers and slowly separating them, creating a string. Good viscosity will produce a string of approximately 1 inch or more before breaking. At lower viscosity, the string will break sooner.

Viscosity should not be assessed on EDTA-preserved synovial fluid, as the preservative will degrade the hyaluronic acid. Ideally, viscosity should be assessed on a fresh sample; however, it can still be assessed confidently using heparin if an anticoagulant is needed.

Cerebrospinal fluid

Normal cerebrospinal fluid (CSF) is of very low cellularity, and concentration techniques are needed to visualize cellular structures microscopically (Table 7.5).

Microscopic evaluation of inflammatory samples

Inflammation is a normal response to infection or tissue damage. Inflammation causes the movement of the inflammatory cells to the area of concern, and by evaluating their numbers and morphologies, the type of inflammation can be determined (Table 7.6). Inflammation can be categorized as suppurative (purulent) (Figure 7.15), granulomatous, pyogranulomatous (Figure 7.16), or eosinophilic (Figure 7.17).

In addition to identifying the inflammatory cell types and their proportions, neutrophil morphology should also be assessed.

Neutrophil pyknosis (Figure 7.18) represents the slow aging and eventual death of the neutrophil. The pyknotic nucleus is dark and condensed. The nucleus may also fragment (karyorrhexis).

Neutrophil karyolysis represents rapid cell death and may also be referred to as "degenerative" (Figure 7.19). It is often seen in septic inflammatory samples where phagocytosed bacteria are noted. The nuclear membrane disintegrates and results in a light-staining, "fluffy" appearance due to the loose chromatin. Cells (neutrophils and macrophages) should be examined closely for evidence of phagocytosed microorganisms (Figure 7.20). Macrophages may phagocytize dead neutrophils or erythrocytes.

Table 7.6 Categories of Inflammation

Suppurative (purulent) = active inflammation	Granulomatous = chronic inflammation	Pyogranulomatous = chronic active inflammation	Eosinophilic
• >85% neutrophils • Nondegenerate neutrophils: appear similarly to the neutrophils seen in blood samples • Degenerative neutrophils: occurs with rapid cell death and displays a lack of an intact nuclear membrane (karyolysis) (Figure 7.15)	• Macrophages are the predominant cell type (>50% of the TNCC) • Typically multinucleated	• A mixture of neutrophils (typically nonde-generative) and macrophages (15–50%). • May also see lymphocytes in low numbers (Figure 7.16)	• Inflammation with 10%–20% eosinophils • Mixture of other cell types included (Figure 7.17)

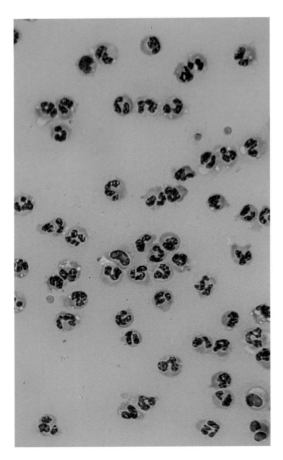

Figure 7.15   Suppurative inflammation.

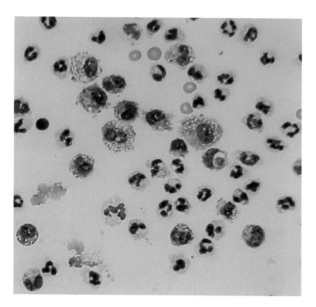

Figure 7.16   Pyogranulomatous inflammation. A mixed population of neutrophils and macrophages is present.

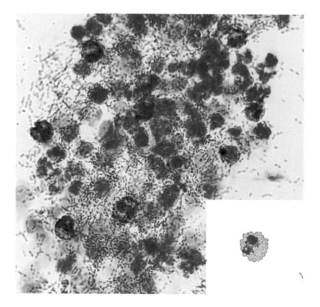

Figure 7.17   An example of eosinophilic inflammation. Numerous bacteria are also present, along with neutrophils. (Inset) Clear view of the eosinophil (equine sample).

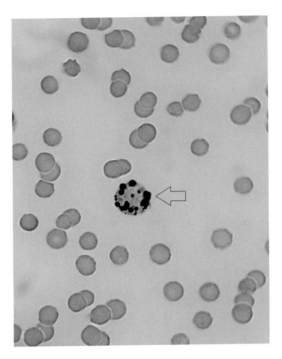

Figure 7.18   Pyknotic neutrophil displaying karyorrhexis.

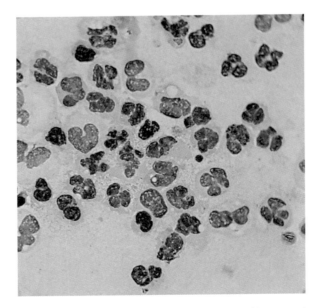

Figure 7.19   Neutrophil karyolysis from a suppurative inflammation sample.

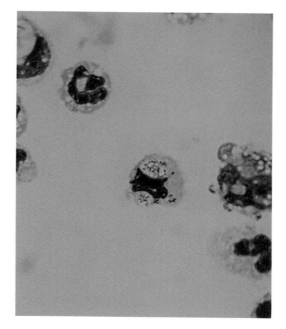

Figure 7.20   Phagocytosed bacteria.

Table 7.7   Criteria of malignancy

Criteria	Microscopic description
Macrokaryosis	Increased nuclear size
Increased nucleus-to-cytoplasm ratio	>1:2 is indicative of malignancy Normal ratio is 1:3 to 1:8
Anisokaryosis	Variation in nuclear size
Multinucleation	Multiple nuclei within a cell (Figure 7.21)
Increased mitotic figures	Increased incidences of mitosis is an abnormal finding in normal tissue (Figure 7.22)
Nuclear molding	Nuclei are molded and misshapen by other nuclei within the cell or a neighboring cell.
Anisonucleosis	Variations in the size or shape of nucleoli (Figure 7.23)
Angular nucleoli	Nucleoli are angular rather than round

Tissue cytology assessment

Following the collection of cells from a mass, the microscopic evaluation should consist of determining the primary cell type, observing the presence of malignant characteristics, and evaluating for signs of an inflammatory process.

Neoplasia and malignancy

Neoplastic samples, unlike inflammatory samples, consist of a homogenous population of a single cell type. These cells can be further evaluated for malignant characteristics (Table 7.7). It should be noted that a concurrent inflammatory process may be present along with neoplasia.

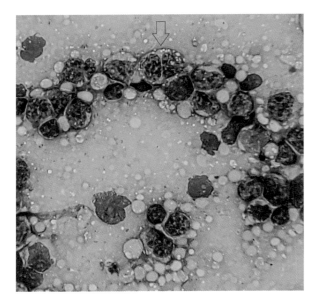

Figure 7.21   Multinucleation (arrow).

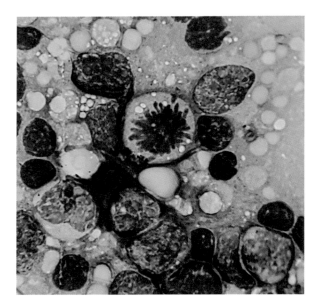

Figure 7.22   Mitotic figure.

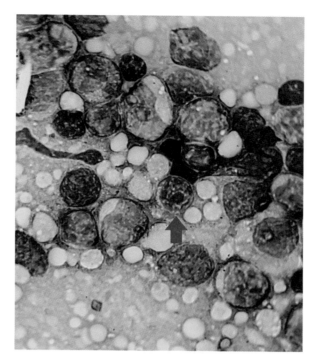

Figure 7.23   Anisonucleosis (arrow).

Table 7.8   Primary cell types

Primary cell type	Characteristics	Terminology
Epithelial (Figure 7.24)	Highly cellular Exfoliate in clumps Cells are large	Benign: adenomas Malignant: carcinomas
Mesenchymal (Figure 7.25)	Less cellular Exfoliate singly Small to medium sized Possess wispy spindles	Benign: -omas (e.g., lipomas) Malignant: sarcomas
Discrete round cell (Figures 7.26)	Highly cellular Exfoliate singly Small to medium sized	Histiocytomas; lymphomas; mast cell tumors; plasma cell tumors; transmissible venereal tumors

Primary cell types

Neoplastic samples can be further evaluated to determine their cell type of origin (Table 7.8). Three common categories include epithelial cell tumors, mesenchymal cell tumors, and discrete round cell tumors.

Lymph node cytology

Lymph node cytology is assessed in cases of lymph node enlargement, and samples are typically obtained using the fine-needle biopsy technique. It serves to differentiate between an inflammatory process, reactive lymph nodes, lymph node hyperplasia, lymphoma, and metastatic neoplasia (Table 7.9).

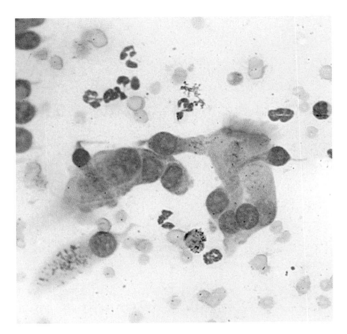

Figure 7.24 Ciliated epithelial cell (from Hendrix CM, Sirois M, *Laboratory Procedures for Veterinary Technicians*, 5th ed. St. Louis, MO: Mosby-Elsevier, 2007).

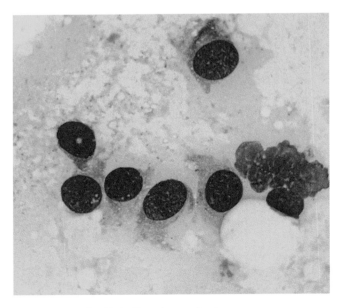

Figure 7.25 Mesenchymal cells. Note the wispy cytoplasms.

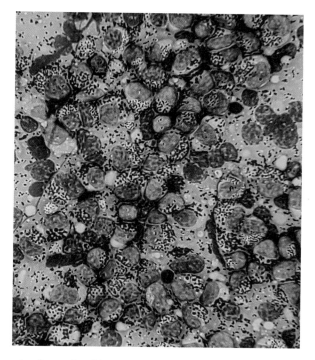

Figure 7.26 Example of round cell types (mast cells from a mast cell tumor).

Table 7.9 Lymph node cytology

Cytology	Cell types seen
Normal lymph node cytology	Small, mature lymphocytes predominate (75–90%) Few intermediate lymphocytes (5–10%) Lymphoblasts (<5%)
Reactive lymph nodes (hyperplasia)	Small, mature lymphocytes Increased numbers of intermediate lymphocytes and lymphoblasts Plasma cells present
Lymphadenitis (inflammation)	Inflammatory cells are present Proportions of inflammatory cells can determine the category of inflammation
Lymphoma (primary neoplasia)	Lymphoblasts >50% Malignant characteristics are noted
Metastatic neoplasia	Homogenous, non-lymph node cells displaying malignant features. Cells could be mesenchymal, epithelial, or round cell in origin.

Ear cytology

Swabs collected from the ear canal can assist in the diagnosis of otitis externa and identify the causative pathogen (Table 7.10). Evaluation consists of examining for the presence of bacteria, typically *Staphylococcus* spp. (cocci) or *Pseudomonas*

Table 7.10 Ear cytology findings

Condition	Microscopic findings
Normal ear cytology	Cornified squamous epithelial cells Very few microorganisms
Otitis externa	Increased numbers of epithelial cells Bacteria or yeast organisms present (Figure 7.27) Possibly inflammatory cells and red blood cells May also include evidence of self-trauma due to excessive scratching
Ear mites	*Otodectes cynotis* parasites and ova (Figure 7.28)

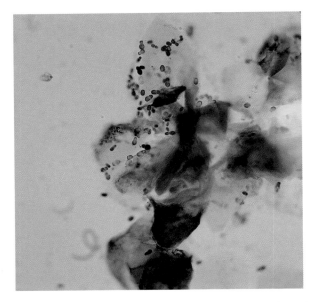

Figure 7.27   Epithelial cells and peanut-shaped *Malassezia* sp. organisms from an ear swab.

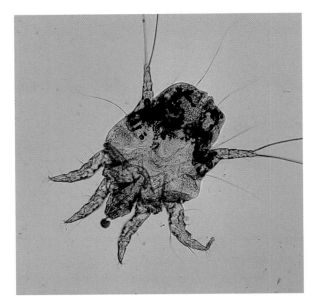

Figure 7.28   *Otodectes cynotis* (ear mite) from a feline ear swab.

(bacilli). Gram staining the slide can assist in more specific bacterial identification. Otitis may also be caused by yeasts of the genus *Malassezia*, which is identified by observing the characteristic budding, dark-staining organism.

Parasitic infestation by *Otodectes cynotis* (ear mite) can also be diagnosed with ear swab collections.

Collection and sample prep

Samples are collected from the external ear canal using the swab technique. If cytological examination is required, the sample is air dried and stained using Romanowsky-type stains or Gram stains. If parasites are suspected, adding the sample to a drop of mineral oil on the slide is all that is required.

Both ears should be thoroughly examined, and slides should be labelled to indicate right versus left.

Canine vaginal cytology

Vaginal cytology can be a useful tool for canine reproduction by determining the stage of estrus of the patient. The hormonal changes occurring in the bitch's estrous cycle influence the proliferation of the vaginal epithelium. By collecting these exfoliated cells and identifying the types and proportions seen, the stage of estrus can be determined with a fair amount of confidence.

Cytological observations should be interpreted along with physical and behavior changes; however, it should be noted that these can vary between individuals.

Collection methods

The exfoliated cells can be collected by using the swab method (Procedure 7.15) or the imprint collection method (Procedure 7.16). Each technique has its advantages and disadvantages (Table 7.11).

Procedure 7.15   Vaginal cytology swab collection method

Materials
- Cotton swab
- 0.9% saline
- Speculum or otoscope cone (optional)
- Microscope slides

Procedure
(1) Moisten the cotton swab with 0.9% saline.
(2) Have someone restrain the dog in a standing position. Use one hand under the abdomen to prevent the dog from sitting.
(3) Depending upon preference, some individuals may use a speculum (or an otoscope cone) to avoid contamination with hair or debris.
(4) Insert the swab into the vulva at a steep craniodorsal angle.
(5) After the swab is inserted roughly 1 inch, lower the angle to approximately 45° and continue. Depending upon the size of the dog, the swab would be inserted anywhere from a couple of inches to several inches.

Table 7.11 Comparison of vaginal cytology collection methods

Swab technique		Impression technique	
Advantages	Disadvantages	Advantages	Disadvantages
• Less contamination • Cells collected directly from the vaginal wall	• More invasive • Requires additional personnel for restraint	• Easier to perform without assistance • Non-invasive	• Increased contamination which could make microscopic evaluation more difficult

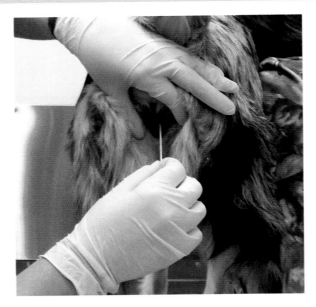

Figure 7.29 Vaginal cytology swab collection method.

(6) Once the swab is inserted, rotate the swab 360° and then remove it. Avoid twisting motions.
(7) Transfer the sample onto the slides as described in Procedure 7.1, "Swab collection method."
(8) Allow to air dry and stain.

Procedure 7.16 Vaginal cytology imprint collection method

Materials
• Microscope slides
• Gauze

Procedure
(1) The dog can be standing, or lying in a ventrodorsal position.
(2) Remove any excess discharge or debris from the vulva using moistened gauze.
(3) Part the vulva and press a slide onto the mucosal surface.
(4) Repeat the imprint 2-3 times.
(5) Allow the slide to air dry and stain.

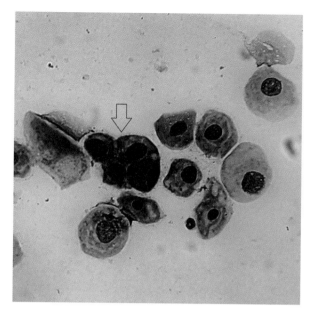

Figure 7.30 Parabasal cells (arrow).

Vaginal cell types

Most of the cells seen microscopically when a vaginal smear is evaluated are vaginal epithelial cells. These cells are present in their various stages of development, and depending upon the stage of estrous, their proportions will vary. These cells are classified as parabasal cells, intermediate cells, and superficial cells. Other microscopic elements that may be seen are neutrophils, red blood cells, bacteria, and a few contaminating cells.

Parabasal cells

Parabasal cells are the smallest of the vaginal epithelial cells. They are round with a high nucleus-to-cytoplasm ratio. They have a greater stain uptake and appear darker than the larger vaginal epithelial cell types (Figure 7.30).

Intermediate cells

Intermediate cells vary in size and shape and can be further classified as small intermediate and large intermediate cells (Figure 7.31). Small intermediate cells retain a round to oval shape with a large nucleus, while large intermediate cells begin to develop an irregular shape with more abundant cytoplasm.

Superficial cells

Superficial cells are the largest vaginal epithelial cells. They are thin and have sharp, angular borders and dark, condensed, pyknotic nuclei (cornification) (Figure 7.32). Superficial cells without a nucleus are referred to as anuclear superficial cells (Figure 7.33). Superficial cells may become folded or rolled up during the collection and slide preparation process.

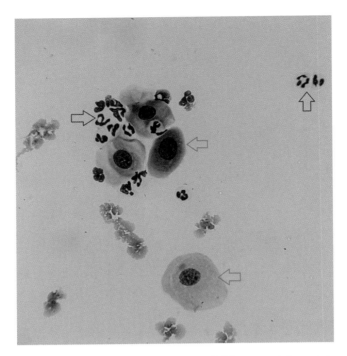

Figure 7.31 Intermediate cells. Small intermediate cell (blue arrow), large intermediate (green arrow). Neutrophils are also present (red arrows).

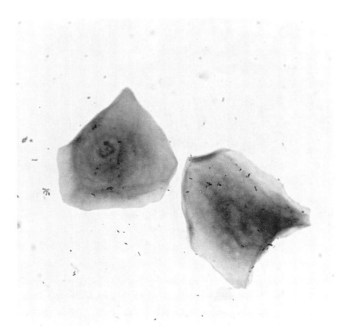

Figure 7.32 Superficial cells with adherent bacteria.

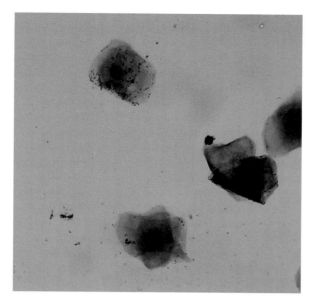

Figure 7.33   Anuclear superficial cells with adherent bacteria.

Stages of estrus

Anestrus
- Duration: 3 to 5 months
- Parabasal and intermediate cells predominate.
- Superficial cells are absent or present in very low numbers.
- Neutrophils may or may not be present.

Proestrus
- Duration: 2 to 15 days
- In early proestrus, parabasal cell numbers begin to decrease as small and large intermediate cells become more common (Figure 7.34).
- In late proestrus, a shift from small intermediate to large intermediate and increased superficial cells begins to occur.
- Red blood cells are usually present.
- Neutrophils and bacteria are present.

Estrus
- Duration: 5 to 17 days
- Cornified superficial cells predominate, with many being anuclear (Figure 7.35).
- Background is clear and free of mucus.
- May or may not contain red blood cells.
- Neutrophils are absent.

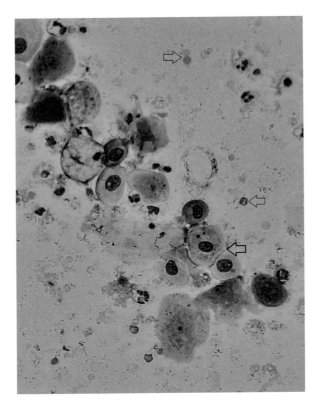

Figure 7.34   Late proestrus. Parabasal cells (green arrows), intermediate cells (black arrow), and a superficial cell (pink arrow). Neutrophils (blue arrows) and RBCs (red arrows) are also present.

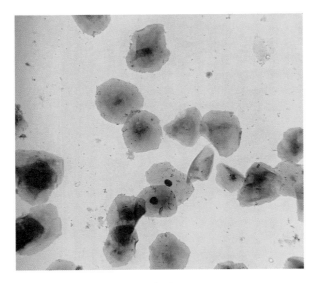

Figure 7.35   Estrus. Superficial cells predominate.

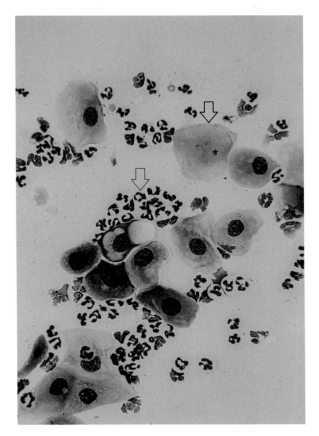

Figure 7.36 Diestrus. Parabasal and small intermediate cells are present. A superficial cell (black arrow) and neutrophils (red arrow) are also present.

Diestrus

- Duration: 2 to 2.5 months
- A dramatic decline in the number of superficial cells is seen.
- Parabasal and small intermediate cells return (Figure 7.36).
- Neutrophils are common, and bacteria are often observed.

Semen evaluation

Evaluating the morphology of spermatozoa in a semen sample is an important part of a comprehensive breeding soundness evaluation. After collection, the quality of a semen sample is determined based upon several characteristics. Volume, concentration, motility, live/dead ratio, and morphology of the sperm are evaluated in conjunction with a physical and behavioral examination of the individual animal. In this section, the focus is on the microscopic evaluation of semen morphology and the live/dead ratio.

Slide preparation

Once the sample has been collected, a smear should be made immediately using a vital dye (Procedure 7.17). An eosin-nigrosin stain is a popular vital dye for this purpose, as it provides a visual discrimination between live and dead spermatozoa (Figure 7.37). This smear can also be used to evaluate morphology.

Procedure 7.17   Semen slide preparation

Materials
- Vital dye (e.g., eosin-nigrosin stain)
- Semen sample
- Microscope slides
  All supplies and samples should be warm

Procedure
(1) Add a small drop of warm stain to a warmed microscope slide.
(2) Mix one drop of semen into the stain.
(3) Gently spread across the slide to make a thin layer using a wooden applicator stick.
(4) Once a smear has been made, the microscopic evaluation can be postponed to a later time.
   Spermatozoa are quite sensitive to cold shock, and if they are exposed to this change in temperature, a higher number of dead spermatozoa will be found. Changes in morphology will also occur.

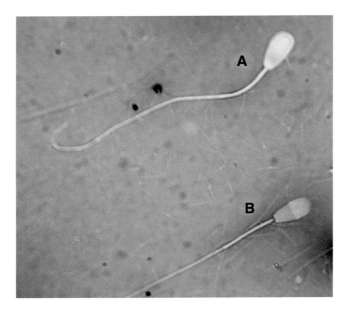

Figure 7.37   Live/dead staining using eosin-nigrosin stain. Live spermatozoa appear white (A). Dead spermatozoa absorb the stain and appear pink (B).

Live/dead ratio

When the eosin-nigrosin stain is used, determination of whether spermatozoa are alive or dead is made by assessing the stain uptake (Figure 7.37). Live sperm resist stain uptake and appear white against the purple-stained background. Dead sperm will take up the stain and will appear pink-purple (similar to the background). Counts are made by examining 100 cells under 400× magnification. Live sperm counts are expressed as a percentage.

Morphology

Sperm morphology can be assessed on the eosin-nigrosin stained slide that was used for the live/dead ratio. The slide is examined under 400× magnification, and the morphology of the spermatozoa is evaluated; spermatozoa with a given morphology are counted and expressed as a percentage of the total.

The anatomy of a spermatozoan cell consists of several structures (Figure 7.38). The cell is composed of a head, acrosome, midpiece, and tail. The tail can be further divided into the principal piece and a terminal piece.

When morphology is evaluated, any abnormalities are classified as either primary or secondary. Primary abnormalities occur during spermatogenesis (Figures 7.39, 7.40, and 7.41), while secondary abnormalities occur at any time

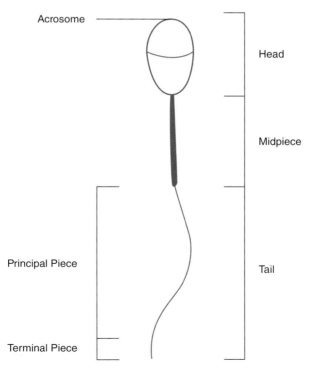

Figure 7.38   Anatomy of a spermatozoan cell.

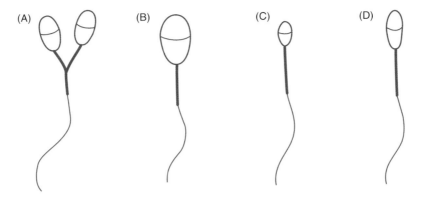

Figure 7.39 Primary cell defects: (A) double head; (B) macrocephalic cell; (C) microcephalic cell; (D) narrow head.

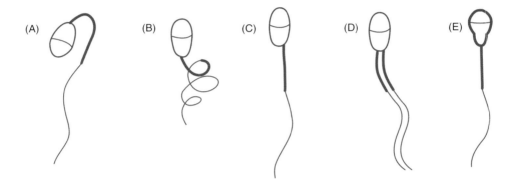

Figure 7.40 Primary cell defects: (A) bent midpiece; (B) coiled midpiece and tail; (C) offset midpiece; (D) double midpiece; (E) pear-shaped head.

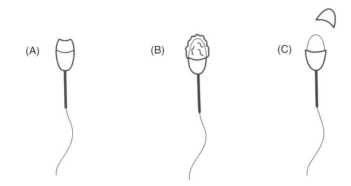

Figure 7.41 Acrosomal defects: (A) knobbed acrosome; (B) ruffled acrosome; (C) loose cap.

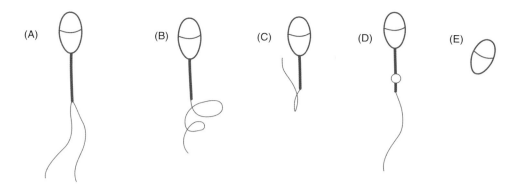

Figure 7.42 Secondary cell defects: (A) double tail; (B) coiled tail; (C) bent tail; (D) protoplasmic droplet; (E) detached head.

between storage in the epididymis to the collection and handling of the specimen. Secondary abnormalities can also occur due to rough handling of the sample or cold shock; therefore, careful sample handling should be a priority. Primary abnormalities are considered more concerning than secondary abnormalities.

Appendix

Temperature conversions

$$°C = (°F - 32) \times \frac{5}{9} \qquad\qquad (A.1)$$

$$°F = \frac{(°C \times 9)}{5} + 32 \qquad\qquad (A.2)$$

Table A.1   Temperature conversions

°C	°F
36.0	96.8
36.5	97.7
37.0	98.6
37.5	99.5
38.0	100.4
38.5	101.3
39.0	102.2
39.5	103.1
40.0	104.0
40.5	104.9
41.0	105.8

Metric conversions

Length
1 m = 39.37 in.
30.48 cm = 1 ft
2.54 cm = 1 in.

Weight
1 kg = 2.2 lbs
1 g = 0.035 oz

Veterinary Technician's Handbook of Laboratory Procedures, Second Edition. Brianne Bellwood and Melissa Andrasik-Catton.
© 2023 John Wiley & Sons, Inc. Published 2023 by John Wiley & Sons, Inc.
Companion website: www.wiley.com/go/bellwoodhandbook2

Volume
3.785 L = 1 gal
0.946 L = 1 quart
29.57 mL = 1 oz
5 mL = 1 teaspoon
15 mL = 1 tablespoon

Metric system

Table A.2   Metric conversions and scientific notation

Factor	Symbol	Prefix
10^{-15}	f	femto
10^{-12}	p	pico
10^{-9}	n	nano
10^{-6}	μ	micro
10^{-3}	m	milli
10^{-2}	c	centi
10^{-1}	d	deci
10	da	deca
10^{2}	h	hecto
10^{3}	k	kilo
10^{6}	M	mega
10^{9}	G	giga
10^{12}	T	tera
10^{15}	P	peta

Glossary

Abdominocentesis	The surgical puncture of the abdomen by a needle to withdraw fluid. Also known as paracentesis.
Accuracy	The closeness of a reading to its true value
Activated partial thromboplastin time (APTT)	A coagulation test used to assess the clotting factors of the intrinsic and common pathways of the coagulation cascade
Agglutination	The formation of aggregates or clumps of red blood cells due to the action of antibodies
Alpha hemolysis	Partial hemolysis that results in a green band or halo around the colonies
Analytic variables	Factors associated with the testing process which could affect the accuracy, precision, and reliability of the test
Anisocytosis	Variation in cell size
Anisokaryosis	Variation in nuclear size
Anisonucleosis	Variation in the size or shape of nucleoli
Antibodies	Proteins produced in response to a specific antigen
Anticoagulant	A substance added to blood which prevents the clotting process
Antigen	A foreign substance which induces an immune response
Anuclear	Lacking a nucleus
Anuria	A lack of urine production.

Veterinary Technician's Handbook of Laboratory Procedures, Second Edition. Brianne Bellwood and Melissa Andrasik-Catton.
© 2023 John Wiley & Sons, Inc. Published 2023 by John Wiley & Sons, Inc.
Companion website: www.wiley.com/go/bellwoodhandbook2

Arthrocentesis	The surgical puncture of a joint by a needle to withdraw fluid
Aseptic	Free from pathogenic organisms
Bacterial spores	Spherical structures produced by some bacteria which are highly resistant to high temperatures, desiccation, and chemical agents.
Beta hemolysis	Complete hemolysis that results in a clear zone surrounding the colonies
Biopsy	The examination of tissue excised from a patient
Broth	Liquid medium which serves to cultivate and maintain profuse growth of microorganisms
Brownian movement	Random movement of microscopic particles in a fluid suspension
Buffy coat	The layer of a packed cell volume which contains the white blood cells and platelets
Capsule	A covering which surrounds some types of bacteria which protects the cell from adverse environmental conditions
Cestodes	Tapeworms
Chromasia	Color of the cell
Cisternal puncture	The surgical puncture of a joint by a needle to withdraw cerebrospinal fluid. Also known as a lumbar puncture.
Complete blood count (CBC)	A group of blood tests used to assess the population and morphologies of erythrocytes, leukocytes, and thrombocytes.
Condenser	A lens system that concentrates (focuses) light into a pencil-shaped cone that passes through the specimen and enters the objective. This allows adjustment of the contrast of the specimen.
Crystalluria	The presence of crystals in the urine
Cylindruria	The presence of casts in the urine
Cystocentesis	A urine collection technique involving the insertion of a needle into the bladder to aspirate a urine sample
Cytokine	A protein which is secreted by certain cells which have an effect on other systems in the body

Definitive host   A host which harbors the adult parasite and in which reproduction occurs

Dermatophytes   Pathogenic fungal organisms which cause ringworm

Differential medium   Medium containing an added indicator used to identify certain types of bacteria based on how they change that indicator

Diopter adjustment   Adjustment that allows focusing of each individual ocular lens. Compensates for differences in right and left vision acuity of the user.

Dysuria   Painful or uncomfortable urination

Ectoparasite   A parasite which lives on or outside the host

ELISA (enzyme-linked immunosorbent assay)   An immunological assay technique in which an enzyme is linked to an antigen or antibody

Endogenous steroids   Naturally occurring steroids produced by the body

Endoparasite   A parasite which lives inside a host

Enriched medium   A general-use medium with added nutrients that meets the growth requirements of most organisms

Erythrocytes   Red blood cells

Exfoliative cytology   The examination of cells which are shed or scraped off the surface of the tissue

Exogenous steroids   Synthetic steroids which are not naturally produced in the body but are administered to the patient

External quality control   Procedures performed by the technician or analyst which evaluate test reliability. These procedures are not automatically performed or built into the equipment.

Fastidious organisms   Organisms with very specific and complex nutritional requirements.

Fibrinogen   A plasma protein that is involved in the clotting process. Under the influence of thrombin, fibrinogen is converted into fibrin. Also know as coagulation factor I.

Fixed-angle centrifuge   A centrifuge which has buckets that are fixed in place and do not swing during operation.

Flagellum   A thin threadlike structure on some bacteria which enables motility

Fungal spores

Fragments which are produced from fungal hyphae which serve a reproductive purpose.

Gamma hemolysis

Absence of hemolysis around the colonies and of change in the appearance of the agar

Hemarthrosis

Bleeding into a joint cavity

Hematocrit

A calculated value which determines the volume of red blood cells as a percentage of whole blood

Hematuria

Presence of intact red blood cells in the urine

Hemoglobinuria

Presence of free hemoglobin in the urine

Hemolysis

Rupture of red blood cells, causing them to release hemoglobin and turn the plasma orange-red

High power

Also known as using the 40x objective lens. With ocular magnification of 10x, the total magnification of high power would be 400x.

HPF

High-power field. One field of view visualized using the 40x objective lens.

Hyphae

Branching filaments of a fungal organism

Hypochromasia

Decreased coloring of the cell

Iatrogenic

Occurring as a result of the activity of the technician (used to describe an error or adverse condition)

Icteric

An increased yellow coloring of the plasma due to higher levels of bile pigments in the blood

Immersion oil

A transparent oil with specific optical characteristics used for microscopy.

Incubator

An enclosed piece of equipment which can provide a controlled environment used for the culturing of microorganisms

Intermediate host

A host that harbors the immature or asexual stage of a parasite

Internal quality control

Procedures automatically or built into the equipment which assess the proper function of the equipment itself

Interpupillary adjustment

An adjustment on the microscope to account for the varying difference in the spacing of the eyes of multiple users

Karyolysis	Disintegration of the cell nucleus occurring with the death of the cell
Karyorrhexis	Fragmentation of a cell nucleus
Kohler illumination	Setting the microscope to align and focus the light. This maximizes both the brightness and uniformity of the specimen.
Left shift	An increase in immature neutrophils
Leukocytes	White blood cells
Lipemia	An increase in lipids in the blood, which result in opaque and white appearance of the plasma
Low power	Also known as using the 10× objective lens. With ocular magnification of 10×, the total magnification of high power would be 100×.
LPF	Low-power field. One field of view visualized using the 10× objective lens.
Lymphopenia	Decreased levels of lymphocytes
Macrocyte	Cell that is larger than is typical for that species
Macrokaryosis	Increased nuclear size
Macroplatelets	Platelets with increased size
Mange	A skin disease caused by parasitic mites.
MCH (mean corpuscular hemoglobin)	Refers to the average weight of hemoglobin within a red blood cell. Expressed in picograms (pg).
MCHC (mean corpuscular hemoglobin concentration)	Refers to the average hemoglobin concentration within a red blood cell. Expressed in grams per liter (g/L).
MCV (mean corpuscular volume)	Refers to the average volume of a red blood cell. Expressed in femtoliters (fL).
Mean platelet volume (MPV)	Refers to the average volume of a platelet. Expressed in femtoliters (fL).
Mesothelial cells	Cells which line the body cavities and internal organs
Metacestode	The larval stage of a tapeworm which is found in an intermediate host

Metastasis	Secondary malignant growths occurring at a distance from the primary site of the cancer
Microcyte	Cell that is smaller than is typical for that species
Microhematocrit centrifuge	A centrifuge used for spinning microhematocrit tubes for packed cell volume measurement
Monocytosis	Increased levels of monocytes
Mycology	The study of fungi
Myiasis	An infection of fly larvae (maggots)
Myoglobin	A protein of skeletal or cardiac muscle origin
Nematodes	Roundworms
Neutropenia	Decreased levels of neutrophils
Neutrophilia	Increased levels of neutrophils
Nucleated RBCs	Immature erythrocytes which retain nuclei, although they are pyknotic
Objective lenses	A series of lenses of a microscope what are nearest to the sample being examined. Each has its own magnification power.
Oliguria	Decreased urine production
Osmosis	The movement of water molecules across a semipermeable membrane to equalize the solute concentrations on both sides
Packed cell volume	A directly measured value obtained by packing red cells through centrifugation and measuring their volume as it compares to the whole blood
Peripheral blood smear	A blood smear made with the goal of producing a monolayer for microscopic evaluation of blood cells
Photometry	The measurement of the intensity or other properties of light which is commonly used in chemistry analyzers
Plasma	The fluid portion of uncoagulated blood
Plateletcrit (PCT)	The volume of whole blood which is occupied by the platelets. Expressed as a percentage.
Poikilocytosis	Presence of abnormally shaped red blood cells

Pollakiuria	Frequent urination
Polychromasia	Increased purple staining of red blood cells, often indicating that the cell is immature
Polymerase chain reactions (PCR)	A reaction used to amplify small pieces of DNA
Polyuria	Increased urine production
Postanalytic variables	Factors occurring posttest which could affect the accuracy, precision, and reliability of the test
Postprandial	After a meal
Preanalytic variables	Factors occurring prior to the testing process which could affect the accuracy, precision, and reliability of the test.
Primary hemostasis	The portion of hemostasis involving the actions of the platelets adhering to and aggregating at the site of injury
Proglottids	A segment of a tapeworm which contains both male and female reproductive organs
Prothrombin time (PT)	A coagulation test used to assess the clotting factors of the extrinsic and common pathways of the coagulation cascade
Pyknosis	The condensing of a cell or nucleus which occurs during apoptosis (natural cell death)
Quality assurance	Procedures or practices which oversee the entire testing process and are designed to minimize errors in increase the reliability of laboratory results
Quantitative	Yielding the quantity or value of the substance being measured
Red cell distribution width (RDW)	A measurement used to indicate the range or variation of cell size in the blood sample
Refractive index	The measurement of the bending of the path of light (refraction)
Refractometer	An instrument used to measure the refractive index of a solution
Reliability	Property of a testing procedure that incorporates both the accuracy and precision of the results produced
Reticulocytes	Immature red blood cells which lack a nucleus

Reticulocytosis	Increased levels of reticulocytes
Rouleaux	A red cell arrangement in which the cells are lined up in row or chains. A common finding in equine blood samples.
Secondary hemostasis	The portion of hemostasis involving the actions of the coagulation factors and the formation of fibrin
Selective medium	Medium that supports the growth of certain microorganisms while inhibiting the growth of others
Sensitivity	A test procedure's ability to detect true positives
Serum	The fluid portion of coagulated blood
Slant	Solid medium contained within a tube and solidified at an angle
Specificity	A test procedure's ability to detect the intended pathogen
Spermatogenesis	Production of spermatozoa
Standard operating procedures	A set of guidelines which outline the method in which all personnel should perform a testing procedure, including the quality assurance and quality control processes
Thoracocentesis	The surgical puncture of the thoracic cavity by a needle to withdraw fluid. Also known as thoracentesis.
Thrombocyte	A platelet
TNCC	Total nucleated cell count
Toxic change	Morphological changes in the neutrophil which occur during maturation as a result of a decrease in maturation time
Trematodes	Flukes
Turbidity	Cloudiness of a fluid due to suspended particles
Urine specific gravity	The concentration and density of a urine sample as it compares to distilled water
Variable-angle centrifuge	A centrifuge with hinged buckets that swing out during operation
Viscosity	A property of a fluid which describes its thickness and stickiness
Zoonosis	A disease which is transmitted from animals to humans

Bibliography

1. Bassert, J. M., Samples, O., Beal, A., McCurnin, D. M., Radin, M. J., and Wellan, M. L. 2018. Hematology and Cytology. In *McCurnin's Clinical Textbook for Veterinary Technicians*, 9th ed., pp. 367-390. Philadelphia: Elsevier Saunders.
2. Bassert, J., Samples, O., Beal, A., McCurnin, D., and Lawhon, S. D. 2018. Clinical Microbiology. In *McCurnin's Clinical Textbook for Veterinary Technicians*, 9th ed., pp. 445-477. Philadelphia: Elsevier Saunders.
3. Bassert, J., Samples, O., Beal, A., McCurnin, D., and Samples, O. M. 2018. Parasitology. In *McCurnin's Clinical Textbook for Veterinary Technicians*, 9th ed., pp. 405-444. Philadelphia: Elsevier Saunders.
4. Bassert, J., Samples, O., Beal, A., McCurnin, D., Radin, M. J., and Wellman, M. L. 2018. Clinical Chemistry, Serology, and Urinalysis. In *McCurnin's Clinical Textbook for Veterinary Technicians*, 9th ed., pp. 391-404. Philadelphia: Elsevier Saunders.
5. Harvey, John W. 2001. *Atlas of Veterinary Hematology*, Philadelphia: W.B. Saunders Company.
6. *Hematology*. eClinpath. 2020. Retrieved March 31, 2022, from https://eclinpath.com/hematology/.
7. *Hemostasis*. eClinpath. 2020. Retrieved March 31, 2022, from https://eclinpath.com/hemostasis/.
8. Hendrix, C. M., and Robinson, E. 2012. Trematodes (Flukes) of Animals and Humans. In *Diagnostic Parasitology for Veterinary Technicians*, 4th ed., pp. 131-142. Maryland Heights: Elsevier Mosby.
9. Hendrix, C. M., Sirois, M., and Martini-Johnson, L. 2007. Urinalysis. In *Laboratory Procedures for Veterinary Technicians*, pp. 151-180. essay. Maryland Heights: Mosby Elsevier.
10. Hendrix, C., and Robinson, E. 2012. Arthropods That Infect and Infest Domestic Animals. In *Diagnostic Parasitology for Veterinary Technicians*, 4th ed., pp. 193-265. Maryland Heights: Elsevier Mosby.
11. Hendrix, C., and Robinson, E. 2012. Common Protozoans That Infect Domestic Animals. In *Diagnostic Parasitology for Veterinary Technicians*, 4th ed., pp. 155-186. Maryland Heights: Elsevier Mosby.
12. Hendrix, C., and Robinson, E. 2022. *Diagnostic Parasitology for Veterinary Technicians*, 5th ed. Maryland Heights: Elsevier Mosby.
13. McCurnin, D. M., Bassert, J. M., and VanSteenhouse, J. L. 2006. Clinical Pathology. In *Clinical textbook for Veterinary technicians*, 6th ed., pp. 203-208. Elsevier Saunders.
14. Rosenfeld, Andrew J., and Dial, Sharon M. 2010. *Clinical Pathology for the Veterinary Team*, Ames: Blackwell Publishing.
15. Sirois, M. 2017. Hematology and Hemostasis. In *Principles and Practice of Veterinary Technology*, pp. 119-149 (essay). Amsterdam: Elsevier.

Veterinary Technician's Handbook of Laboratory Procedures, Second Edition. Brianne Bellwood and Melissa Andrasik-Catton.
© 2023 John Wiley & Sons, Inc. Published 2023 by John Wiley & Sons, Inc.
Companion website: www.wiley.com/go/bellwoodhandbook2

16. Sirois, M. 2020. *Laboratory Procedures for Veterinary Technicians*, 7th ed. Amsterdam: Elsevier.
17. *Specimen collection*. BD. 2022. Retrieved January 31, 2022, from https://www.bd.com/en-ca/offerings/capabilities/specimen-collection
18. Thrall, Mary Anna, Weiser, Glade, Allison, Robin W. and Campbell, Terry W. 2012 *Veterinary Hematology and Clinical Chemistry*, 2nd ed. Ames: Blackwell Publishing.
19. Zajac, A. M., Conboy, G. A., American Association of Veterinary Parasitologists, and ProQuest. 2012. *Veterinary clinical parasitology*, 8th ed. Hoboken: Wiley-Blackwell.

Index

acanthocytes, 32
acarina, 132-137
accuracy, 13, 68, 73
acid-fast (Ziehl-Neelsen) stain, 149-150
ACT *see* activated coagulation time
activated coagulation time (ACT) test, 64
activated partial thromboplastin time (aPTT), 12, 64
agar, 142-146
agglutination, 41-42
ammonium urate, 92
amorphous phosphate, 92
analytic variables, 15
Anaplasma spp., 38
anemia, reticulocyte count, 27-30
anestrus, 195
anisocytosis, 31
anisonucleosis, 185, 187
aPTT *see* activated partial thromboplastin time
arthropods *see* mites
artifacts
  erythrocytes, 42-43
  urine, 96-97
aspiration technique, fine-needle biopsy, 185-186
automated hematology, 65-66

Babesia spp., 38
bacteria
  ear swabs, 189-191
  morphology, 150-155
  urinalysis, 94, 97
  see also microbiology
Baermann technique, 107-108
band neutrophils, morphology, 49, 50-55
Barr bodies, 56, 57
basophil morphology, 49, 51-55
basophilic stippling, 36
bilirubin, 85, 94
biopsies
  centesis, 170-171
  fine-needle, 163-166
  impression smears, 168-169
  punch, 166-167
  scrapings, 169-170
  wedge, 166, 168
bladder expression, 76, 77

blood collection
  order of draw, 70
  parasites, 100
  tubes, 69-70, 100
blood-borne parasites, 127, 128
BMBT *see* buccal mucosal bleeding time test
bovines
  cestodes, 122
  leukocyte morphology, 53-54
  nematodes, 117-119
  protozoans, 124-128
  Rickettsiae, 128
  trematodes, 124
broths, 142
Brownian movement, 155
buccal mucosal bleeding time test (BMBT), 62-63
burr cells, 34
burrowing mites, 133, 139

calcium carbonate, 92
calcium oxalate dihydrate, 93
calcium oxalate monohydrate, 93
calibration, refractometers, 10
cancer, 185-189
canines
  cestodes, 120-121
  estrus, 195-197
  leukocyte morphology, 50-51
  nematodes, 110-114
  protozoans, 124-128
  trematodes, 124
  vaginal cytology, 191-197
capsules, 150
casts, 95-96
catheterization, 76, 77
cell counters, 12
cell inclusions, 35-37
cellophane tape preparation, 99-100
centesis, 170-171
centrifugation, 6-7, 104-105, 173
cerebrospinal fluid (CSF), 181
cestodes (tapeworms), 119-123
  canines, 120-121
  cystic stage, 123
  equines, 122
  felines, 120-121

Veterinary Technician's Handbook of Laboratory Procedures, Second Edition. Brianne Bellwood
and Melissa Andrasik-Catton.
© 2023 John Wiley & Sons, Inc. Published 2023 by John Wiley & Sons, Inc.
Companion website: www.wiley.com/go/bellwoodhandbook2